LUNG INFLAMMATION

Edited by **Kian Chung Ong**

Lung Inflammation
http://dx.doi.org/10.5772/57068
Edited by Kian Chung Ong

Contributors
Masaki Fujita, Stephan Van Eeden, Kunihiko Hiraiwa, Elisa Gomes, Geraint Florida-James, Tobias Stoeger

Published by InTech
Janeza Trdine 9, 51000 Rijeka, Croatia

Publishing Process Manager Iva Lipovic
Technical Editor InTech DTP team
Cover InTech Design team

First published May, 2014
Printed in Croatia

Additional hard copies can be obtained from orders@intechopen.com

Lung Inflammation, Edited by Kian Chung Ong
p. cm.
ISBN 978-953-51-1373-7

For EU product safety concerns:
IN TECH d.o.o., Prolaz Marije Krucifikse Kozulić 3, 51000 Rijeka, Croatia,
info@intechopen.com or visit our website at intechopen.com.

Meet the editor

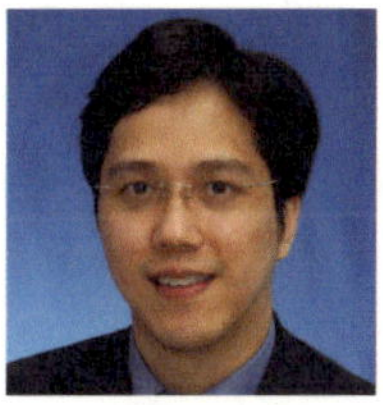

After completing his basic medical education (MBBS) at the National University of Singapore in 1987, Dr. Ong was accepted as a member of the Royal College of Physicians (MRCP) in the United Kingdom in 1993 and subsequently completed his specialist training in Respiratory Medicine at the Singapore General Hospital. In 1996 and 1997, Dr. Ong was a Fellow in the Department of Pulmonary and Critical Care Medicine, Stanford University Medical Center, USA, and was also a visiting clinical and research Fellow in the Stanford Sleep Disorders Clinic and Research Center, USA. Dr. Ong has been a Fellow of the Royal College of Physicians (FRCP) in Edinburgh since 2002. He is also a Fellow of the American College of Chest Physicians (ACCP). Dr. Ong is the President of the Chronic Obstructive Pulmonary Disease Association (Singapore) and is recognized by the Global Initiative for Chronic Obstructive Lung Disease (GOLD) as the National Leader in Singapore. He presently is in private specialist practice at the Mount Elizabeth Medical Centre, Singapore.

Contents

Preface

In order to perform its function in gas exchange, the lungs and all components of the respiratory system are constantly exposed to pathogens, toxins, pollutants, irritants, and allergens in the environment. Lung inflammation involves an array of mechanisms to defend the lung against these extrinsic agents and to repair injured tissue. Additionally, the lungs are a frequent target at risk to conditions associated with systemic inflammation that cause multi-organ damage. The inflammatory reaction in the lung is a complex and dynamic process, and our understanding in this field is rapidly progressing. Further elucidation of the complexity of inflammation will likely improve the clinician's approach to as well as the treatment of a myriad of lung disorders. The chapters in this book are selected topics of current interest in lung inflammation.

Dr. Kian Chung Ong
KC Ong Chest & Medical Clinic
Mount Elizabeth Medical Centre
Singapore

Chapter 1

Lung Inflammation, Oxidative Stress and Air Pollution

Elisa Couto Gomes and Geraint Florida-James

Additional information is available at the end of the chapter

http://dx.doi.org/10.5772/58252

1. Introduction

This is a very relevant chapter in the context of "Lung Inflammation" because it details and discusses an important theme in this area: air pollution. The analyses of epidemiological studies, conducted in various urban centres, have provided coherent evidence that elevated levels of air pollution are associated with an increased risk of respiratory disease and mortality. The whole population is affected, but the active and athletic population is of special concern because of the amount of time they spend training and/or competing outdoors, eliciting high ventilation rates that result in higher pollutants delivery to the lungs.

This chapter addresses the systemic effects that inhaled pollutants have as well as the local pulmonary inflammatory processes and oxidative stress. The consequences that these processes may impose to the health and performance of the active population will also be described. The use of antioxidants to counteract the deleterious oxidative stress of exercise when performed in a polluted environment is discussed here too.

2. Air pollution

Air pollution can be composed by a cocktail of different substances that in large amounts can be harmful to the ecosystem. The industrial revolution marks the beginning of an accelerated global urbanization process. As a result, large urbanized areas suffer from, amongst other problems, a high concentration of air pollutants. The most evident form of air pollution is a dark layer of gas – also known as smog – present above big cities. Nevertheless, there are different kinds of air pollution that are not as visible. Sources include natural processes, such as volcano emissions, and also industrialized sources found in urban centres linked to human activities. The latter includes power plants, factories, burning of fossil fuel and transportation.

2.1. Classification of air pollutants

Air pollutants can be found in different forms and sizes. They can be solid particles, liquid molecules or gases. According to the way they are generated these pollutants can be considered as primary (directly produced) or secondary (formed by the interaction of primary pollutants). Some pollutants can be both produced directly as well as formed by the reaction of other pollutants. In addition, there are indoor and outdoor pollutants, all of which can be detrimental to human health. Although indoor pollution is generally low, its levels can be augmented by the use of several chemical products (e.g. cleaning products, paints), heaters, stoves and indoor smoking. Fortunately, various countries have already adopted policies that ban smoking in closed public spaces. Description and classification of the main pollutants resulting from human activity are listed in table 1 below.

Air Pollutant	Characteristics	Source
Ammonia (NH_3)	• Gas • No colour • Strong pungent smell	Produced industrially. Mostly used as fertiliser to agricultural crops (over 80%). Also used, for example, in the fermentation and textile industry, as cleaning product, and as antimicrobial agent for food products.
Carbon monoxide (CO)	• Gas • No colour • No smell	A major source of this poisonous gas is vehicular exhaust. It is also a product of incomplete combustion of carbon-containing fuels.
Nitrogen dioxides (NO_2)	• Gas • Brownish-red colour • Strong smell	Released by internal combustion engines and power-plants. Indoor sources of this pollutant include gas and kerosene heaters. It is also released by electric discharge during storms. NO_2 is also a precursor for the formation of O_3 pollution.
Ozone (O_3) or Tropospheric O_3 or ground level O_3	• Gas • No colour • Strong smell	This highly oxidant pollutant is formed by the reaction of nitrogen oxides and volatile organic compounds in the presence of sunlight. As it is easily transported by the wind it can be found in high concentrations not only in large urban areas but also in rural areas.
Particulate Matter (PM)	• Solid or liquid particles	This pollutant can vary in size, form and composition being made up by a mixture of extremely small particles (metals, soil, dust) and liquid droplets (acids, organic compounds). The smaller the PM size the deeper it can penetrate into the lungs and might even be able to pass to the systemic circulation and affect other organs.
Sulfur oxides (SOx)	• Gas • No colour • Strong smell	Amongst the highly reactive gases of this group is the sulphur dioxide (SO_2) that is produced by the burning of fuels such as petrol, diesel, and coal. It is naturally released into the atmosphere by activated volcanoes.
Volatile Organic Compounds (VOCs)	• Gases emitted from solids and liquids • Strong smell	VOCs are mainly indoor pollutants because they can be released by a variety of materials and products which are used in the households and offices such as paints, disinfectant, air-fresheners and photocopy machines. VOCs are also released by fuels. As mentioned previously they are precursors of O_3.

Table 1. Main primary pollutants resulting from human activity

3. General health consequences of exposure to air pollution

The analyses of recent epidemiological studies, conducted in various urban centres, have provided coherent evidence that elevated levels of air pollution are associated with an increased risk of respiratory diseases, chronic obstructive lung diseases (COPD), cancers, cerebrovascular-strokes, cardiovascular diseases and mortality. These occur due to the nature of the pollutants and via their impacts on the respiratory and cardiovascular systems [1-7]. Air pollution does not only affect individuals that are directly exposed to it, but it also has a deleterious effect on foetal development and preterm birth. Various studies have shown that decreases in neonate birth weight are associated with exposure to air pollution [8-10]. Children are also very susceptible to the harmful effects of pollution exposure. This is reflected by an increase in the number of young children admitted to hospitals for acute lower respiratory infection: pneumonia and bronchiolitis. These respiratory infections are the largest causes of mortality among young children worldwide, especially in developing countries. Within these countries a low socioeconomic status potentiates the consequences of air pollution exposure [5, 11, 12].

These adverse effects on health, caused by air pollution, have been shown to occur in both developed and developing countries. However, its health-related burden falls most heavily on developing countries [3, 6, 13-15]. According to the World Health Organisation [16], air pollution is responsible for over 800, 000 premature deaths each year, with more than 6 million years of life lost annually. Asia alone would account for approximately two thirds of these numbers [2]. It goes without saying that this air pollution disease-burden is a great economic issue to countries affected [14].

The World Health Organisation, together with governments of various countries, have proposed guidelines for maximum concentrations of the different pollutants (see table 2). Nevertheless, this does not always translate into national policies and various cities are unable to maintain pollution levels within the suggested guidelines. The implementation of anti-pollution measures is not always straight forward. At times, for example, it means there is a need to change energy sources and invest in green technology. As a consequence, some countries are more reluctant than other to execute such measures [3, 17].

In relation to indoor air pollutants, on March 2004, the Republic of Ireland became the first country to completely ban smoking from workplaces. More and more countries gradually adopted this public-space smoking ban. Nowadays, most countries in the world have some kind of law pertaining to the issue. There is a growing body of evidence on the positive health outcomes and the economic benefits related to the adoption of smoke-free laws. Improvements in lung function, airway and systemic inflammation, and adverse respiratory symptoms were observed in individuals working in bars [18, 19]. Hospital admissions of children and adults presenting asthma and other pulmonary illnesses also decreased as a result of reduced exposure to environmental tobacco smoke [20-22]. Smoking bans also positively impacted individuals with heart diseases which include myocardial infarction, unstable angina and stroke [20, 22-24].

Pollutant	Averaging time	Air quality guideline values (ug/m^3)
PM2.5	1year	10
	24 h (99th percentile)	25
PM10	1year	20
	24 h (99th percentile)	50
O_3	8 h, daily maximum	100
NO_2	1year	40
	1 h	200
SO_2	24 h	20
	10 min	500
Source: (WHO 2012)		

Table 2. Updated WHO air guideline values

4. Oxidative stress and air pollution

The mechanism responsible for the adverse effect of oxidant pollutants – ozone, PM – in the lungs, which might possibly also lead to a systemic outcome, would be its direct and indirect oxidative reaction with molecules and cells present in the airways [25, 26]. This might result in oxidative stress in the airway tissues [27]. But what is oxidative stress?

4.1. Oxidative stress

Oxidative stress can be defined as damage that might occur in cell components, such as membranes, RNAs and DNA, as a result from an imbalance in the body's ability to neutralize certain molecules or to repair the resulting damage. Free radicals and reactive species (reactive oxygen species and reactive nitrogen species) are molecules that easily react with other molecules to become more stable. This is an oxidation reaction, because there is transfer of electrons from a substance to the free radicals/reactive species (oxidaizing agents). When in our organism these reactions occur with cell components, which could have detrimental effects such as cell function impairment and cell death. Nevertheless, the body has an elaborate antioxidant defence system that neutralizes the reactive species and free radicals so as to maintain a redox homeostasis. This balance, however, can be disturbed if the concentration of pro-oxidants (reactive species and free radicals) overwhelms the available antioxidants or if the antioxidants are depleted due to disease or poor diet. This associated with reduced repairing process, can result in oxidative stress, and impaired cellular function may occur. In humans, oxidative stress has been shown to be the cause and consequence of various diseases (Fig 1). These include, but are not limited to, cancers, atherosclerosis, Alzheimer's disease, Parkinson's disease, dementia, heart diseases and pulmonary disorders [28-30].

http://dx.doi.org/10.5772/58252

On the other hand, free radicals and reactive species are essential to our well-being. This happens because these molecules are necessary for a variety of reactions to occur. For example, they are used by the immune system to attack and kill pathogens in a process called respiratory burst. They are also used for gene stimulation, cell signalling, vasoregulation and inflammatory processes [31, 32].

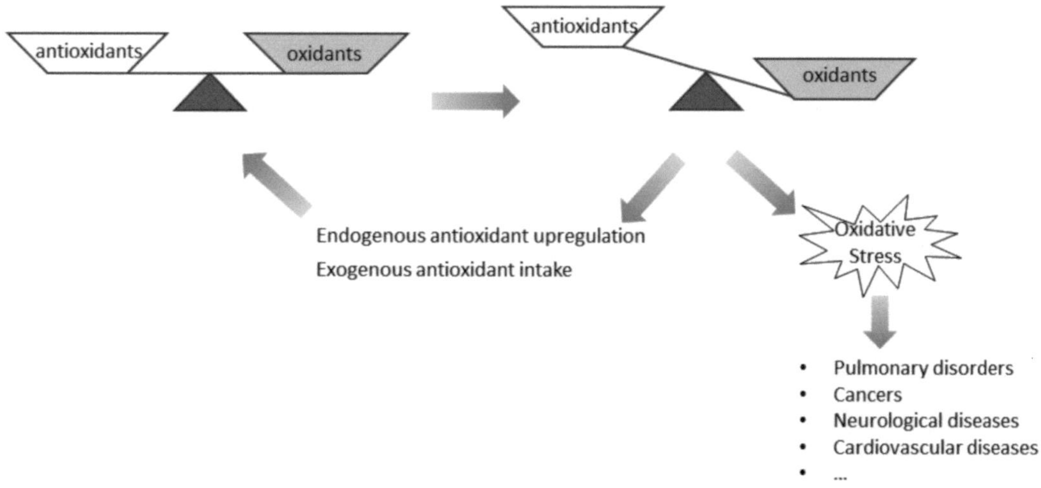

Figure 1. Redox balance

4.2. Antioxidants

Antioxidants are often reducing agents capable of being promptly oxidized by free radicals and reactive species, eliminating their pro-oxidant nature before they react with cell components. There is a wide range of antioxidants in body fluids, tissues and organs. They are present both intracellular and extracellular, working synergistically in a network to balance the free radicals and reactive species. Therefore, the action of one antioxidant may depend on the correct function of other antioxidants in the system.

Antioxidants are both synthesized *in vivo* and absorbed through the diet and they can be divided into two groups: enzymatic and non-enzymatic. Enzymatic antioxidants include superoxide dismutase (SOD), glutathione peroxidase (GPX) and catalase (CAT). Each of these enzymes is responsible for the reduction of different pro-oxidants and they are located in different cellular compartments. Glutathione, vitamin C, vitamin E, carotenoids, and uric acid are some examples of non-enzymatic antioxidants. Similarly to the enzymatic antioxidant, these are present in different cellular compartments and elicit distinct antioxidant properties which maximize their effectiveness [29]. Antioxidants can also be classified according to their soluble nature: hydrophilic (water soluble) or lipophilic (lipid soluble). It is this characteristic that allows them to be present in different parts of the cells.

Antioxidant	Solubility	Concentration in human serum (μM)
Glutathione	Hydrophilic	4
Lipoic acid	Hydrophilic	0.1-0.7
Melatonin	Hydrophilic and lipophilic	Varies throughout the day
Ubiquinol (coenzyme Q)	Lipophilic	5
Uric acid	Hydrophilic	200-400
Vitamin A (retinol)	Lipophilic	1-3
Vitamin C (ascorbic acid)	Hydrophilic	50-60
Vitamin E (α-tocopherol)	Lipophilic	10-40
β-carotene	Lipophilic	0.5-1

Table 3. Important antioxidants

Most antioxidants undergo redox cycling. This means that once oxidized they can be reduced to their former state and act again as an antioxidant. Nevertheless, this redox cycling allows the antioxidant to act as pro-oxidant promoting free radical formation. This would happen if there is an unbalance in the antioxidant network system. Vitamin C and vitamin E are examples of antioxidants with this characteristic, while melatonin is considered a terminal antioxidant because it cannot be recycled.

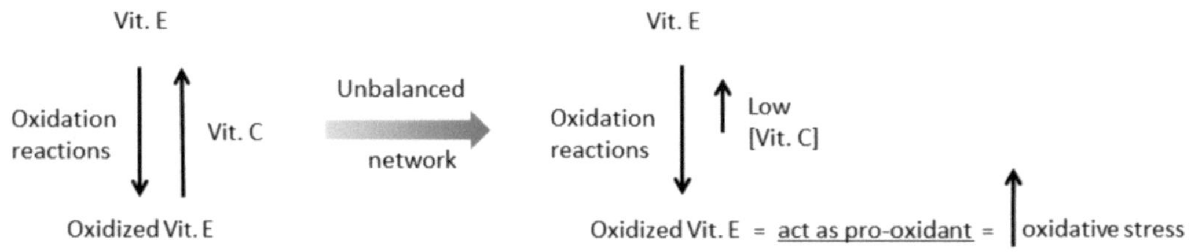

Figure 2. Redox cycling of vitamin E (vit E) by vitamin C (Vit. C)

4.3. Lung oxidative stress

Oxidant air pollutants such as ozone, particulate matter and nitrogen dioxide have been shown to induce lung inflammation through stimulation of the oxidative stress process. Little is known, however, about their effects as oxidant compounds in the lungs or about the role and the effectiveness of the antioxidants present in the respiratory tract lining fluid (RTLF) in scavenging and protecting against their harmful effects. A great variety of antioxidants can be found in human RTLF. Their concentration and distribution throughout the airways, however, is not homogeneous, with high levels of GSH in the alveolar epithelial regions and uric acid predominating in the upper airways [33, 34].

Numerous studies have investigated the effects by which O_3 affects the human lungs. Nevertheless, the mechanisms responsible for such adverse effects, such as an increase in the airway inflammation and impairment in lung function, are only partly understood. It is known that when O_3, or indeed any gas, is inhaled, it first comes into contact with the RTLF. Indeed, ozone is not able to infiltrate further than the RTLF and the membranes of cells from the lung-air interface, yet it is still known to cause damage beyond the lungs. Once O_3 comes into contact with the RTLF, it induces oxidative stress by two different mechanisms. The first would be by reacting directly with the constituents of the RTLF and the underlying epithelium [26]. It has been suggested that antioxidants present in the RTLF, such as glutathione, uric acid and ascorbic acid have an important role in neutralizing part of the radical generation, hence reducing the ozone induced oxidative stress [35]. Studies analysing the effect of ozone inhalation and airway antioxidant consumption have indeed shown significant alterations in airway antioxidants, such as uric acid, ascorbic acid and GSH [36-38].

The second mechanism by which ozone can increase the oxidation process is indirectly because, even though O_3 does not react directly with the epithelial cells, these cells do react in response to the oxidation products produced in the RTLF. As a consequence they release a variety of pro-inflammatory mediators and more reactive species [25, 26]. These processes combined could overwhelm the local and systemic antioxidant network leading to an increase in the oxidative process, the intensity of which varies depending on the O_3 inhaled dose and also on the antioxidants present in the lining fluid. If the oxidative stress is sufficient, the activation of an inflammatory response occurs and is characterized by the intense arrival and activation of neutrophils. These neutrophils produce further ROS through the respiratory burst process. Hence, the overproduction of ROS might result in oxidative stress in the airway tissues. The hypothesis is that the antioxidants present in the epithelial lining fluid of the lungs would neutralize the excess production of free radicals and ROS, consequently reducing lung injury induced by air pollution [27, 35]. This will be discussed in the following sections.

5. Lung inflammation and air pollution

Airway inflammation and any other inflamed tissue can be characterized by an increase in inflammatory cells, such as neutrophils and macrophages, as well as inflammatory mediators: interleukin-6 (IL-6), interleukin-8 (IL-8), and prostaglandins. An increase in neutrophil numbers and percentage is a good indicator of the beginning of an inflammatory response because these cells account for 50-60% of the total white blood cells in the circulation and are the first cell type to migrate to sites of injury and inflammation. When a tissue is inflamed, an increase in the expression of adhesion molecules of the selectin family (E-and P-selectin molecules) occurs in the local endothelium. This process is mediated by cytokines and other inflammatory mediators. Neutrophils present in the blood recognise the site of inflammation because of these adhesion molecules which bind to the other molecules (mucin-like cell-adhesion molecules, CAM) on the neutrophil surface. This step is referred to as rolling: the first step to the attachment of neutrophils onto the endothelium. In order for them to adhere firmly and be able to migrate through the endothelial to the inflamed site, the neutrophils are activated by various chemoattractants derived from epithelial cells exposed to a foreign body, IL-8 being an important one. Once the adhesion processes is successful the neutrophils can initiate their transendothelium migration. Upon arrival at the inflamed tissue, neutrophils release a number of chemoattractants to amplify the inflammatory response by recruiting other cells.

The cytokine IL-8 is a mediator of the immune function and helps regulate the immune response. It is secreted by a variety of cells, including neutrophils, macrophages and endothelial cells, and is a chemotactic for cells such as neutrophils and T cells. In addition, it has been linked to a wide variety of pathologic conditions characterized by an increase in neutrophil count. Thus, an increase in IL-8 levels is linked to an increase in neutrophils [39]. IL-6 is another important mediator in the development of an inflammatory process. It is produced mainly by T-cells and macrophages; and, together with IL-1 and TNF-α, stimulate both local and systemic changes of an inflammatory response. This cytokine – IL-6 – has been thoroughly studied in immunological responses to exercise [40-41].

Inhalation of air pollution has been shown to stimulate airway inflammation due to its oxidative nature. Airway inflammation can be detected by both a local increase in inflammatory cells as well as inflammatory mediators. The depletion of antioxidants found in the airways, characterizes the oxidative process that triggers an inflammatory response due to epithelial damage [42, 43]. Both the inflammatory mediators and the antioxidants can be measured using different techniques, each with its own advantages and disadvantages. Bronchial biopsies and brochoalveolar lavage (BAL) are quite invasive procedures that require local anesthesia and need to be performed in a medical environment [44]. These two techniques have the advantages of sampling the more distal regions of the airway and the biopsies retrieves tissue samples which can give further information about the local inflammatory process. The sputum induction procedure and the nasal lavage (NL) procedure, on the other hand, are less invasive and less technically difficult procedures than the previously-mentioned bronchial techniques and can be repeated at multiple time points [37, 45]. Sputum induction and NL are techniques that sample the upper respiratory airways.

There has been a variety of studies analysing airway inflammation of individuals exposed to O_3 pollution. Due to the similar oxidative nature of O_3 in relation to other pollutants, the results of these studies can be, in a certain way, generalized to include them too. Nevertheless, when analysing the literature, it is always essential to take into account the total volume of pollutants inspired by the participants, as well as the techniques used to sample the airway compartments. Ideally it would also be relevant to take into account the antioxidant concentrations in the RTLF, which has been shown to vary between individuals. In order to increase the amount of air – and consequently air pollution – inspired in a shorter amount of time, most studies use exercise protocols in association with the exposure.

Airway inflammation can lead to the destruction of the cilia of the epithelial cells that line the respiratory tract. The cilia have an important immune function because they constantly move the mucus up from the lungs to the back of the throat where it is eliminated or swallowed and digested. The mucus serves as a "trap" to infectious agents and small particles, such as pollutants and allergens, preventing them to enter deep into the airways. Gas pollutants are

http://dx.doi.org/10.5772/58252

not trapped in the mucus, though they can exacerbate its production and destroy the cilia making the airways more susceptible to the invasion of other foreign agents. Another consequence of airway inflammation is lung epithelial injury which leads to an open interface between the lung and the blood. This facilitates the dispersion of microbes to the rest of the body, initiating a systemic inflammatory response. If the lung epithelial injury is chronic and the tissue is recurrently going through a repairing process, this can lead to fibrosis with consequential decrease in lung function, chest discomfort, fatigue and weakness.

Injury and toxicity involving the respiratory epithelium can be assessed by a simple and noninvasive way by measuring the concentration of Clara cell protein, also known as CC16, CC10 or Uteroglobin. This protein is secreted, as the name indicates, by Clara cells. The function of these cells is mainly the protection of the respiratory tract. They present a high content of xenobiotic metabolizing enzymes which protect our system against inhaled particles including pollutants [46, 47]. CC16 is a small protein with an important role in decreasing the inflammation of the respiratory tract and protecting it against the harmful effects of oxidative stress [48]. This protein can be measured by the methods used to assess the respiratory airways, including the NL procedure. In addition, CC16 can also be found in the blood, where it is derived almost exclusively from the airways [46]. In normal healthy individuals, the serum level of CC16 ranges, on average, from 10 to 15 $ug \cdot l^{-1}$ [49]. Yet, the concentration of this protein in the blood has been shown to rise as a result of pulmonary inflammation and increases in the permeability of the lung epithelial barrier. The lung–blood barrier offers some resistance to the bi-directional movement of large proteins such as albumin. Nevertheless, the high concentration of CC16 in the respiratory tract secretions and its small size permit its diffusion into the blood [50, 51] where it can easily be detected by conventional enzyme immunoassays [52].

The bi-directional exchange of proteins between lung and blood is regulated by several factors, such as the size of the proteins, the epithelium permeability and the driving force of the transepithelial concentration gradient. The concentration gradient allows the movement of proteins from an area of high concentration to an area of low concentration. In the case of CC16, this if from the lung to the blood; but albumin, for example, moves in the opposite direction. The large difference between the concentration gradients can be related to the difference in the compartment sizes in which the proteins are diluted. The concentration gradient is also influenced by the removal of the protein from the compartment into which it is leaking-proteins that enter the lung interstitium are rapidly cleared by lymphatic drainage [51].

The changes that occur in serum concentrations of CC16 may result from three different mechanisms. The first mechanism would result from the increase in the permeability of the lung epithelial barrier, and this has as a consequence a higher diffusion of CC16 into the blood. This can happen following exposure to ozone, which causes epithelial lung injury, or more specifically, damage to the tight junctions of the cells (fig. 4) [51, 53]. A second possibility is the decrease or increase in the production or secretion of CC16 from the Clara cells present in the respiratory tract. A reduction in the number of Clara cells has been shown to occur following chronic exposure to lung toxicants such as silica particles [54]. The third mechanism that would lead to an enhancement in the levels of serum CC16 would result from a reduction in the clearance of this protein by the kidney. Serum CC16 has a half-life of approximately 2-3

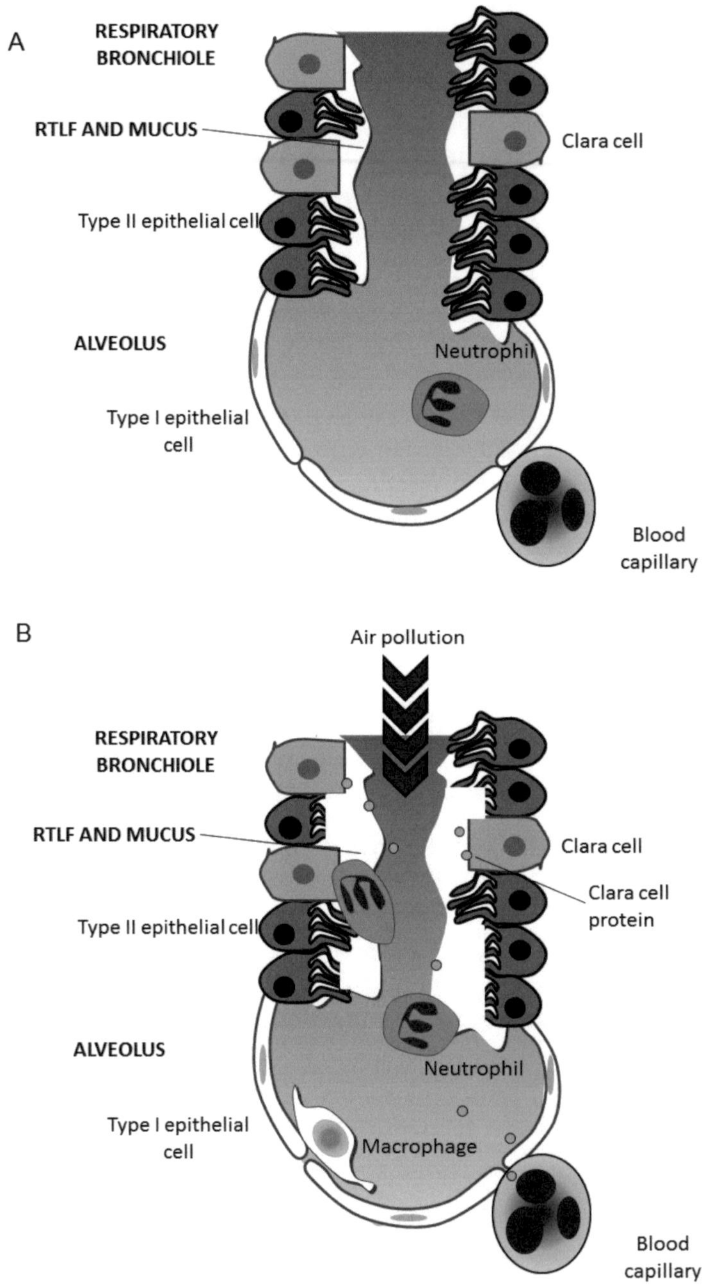

Figure 3. Respiratory bronchiole before (A) and after (B) air pollution exposure.

h due to its rapid clearance through the kidney [46]. Hence, the variation in CC16 serum levels can only be used as a specific biomarker of the airway epithelium integrity if the individual does not present renal dysfunction.

http://dx.doi.org/10.5772/58252

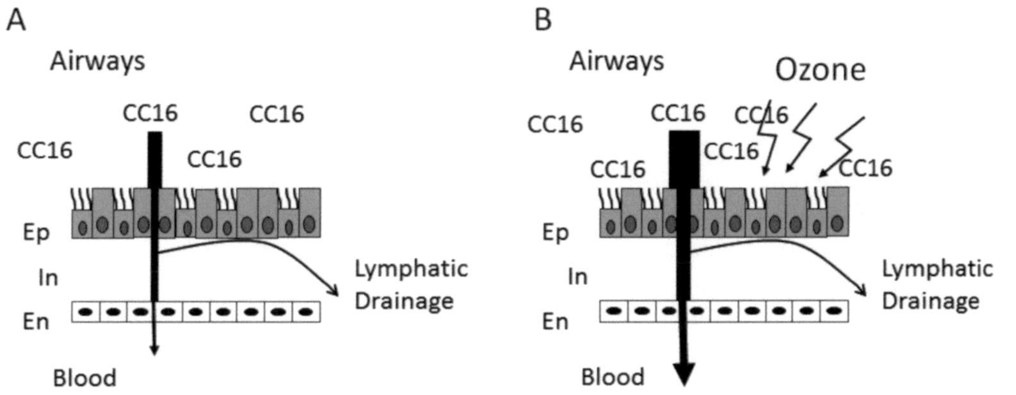

Figure 4. Movement of CC16 from the airways to the blood. (A) Under normal conditions, (B) after exposure to ozone. The thickness of the arrows is used to illustrate the relative permeability of the different barriers and the increase in the CC16 flux after ozone exposure. Abbreviations: Ep – epithelium; In-interstitium; En – endothelium (adapted from Broeckaert *et al.* 2000b).

Both acute and chronic exposure to toxicants has been shown to elicit changes in serum CC16 levels. This supports the theory that this protein is a sensitive and suitable biomarker of lung injury [46, 54]. A study conducted with firefighters [55] showed that acute smoke inhalation significantly increased serum CC16 levels. In addition to smoke inhalation, the firefighters also had to perform physically demanding tasks. Serum CC16 concentration was measured immediately after exposure and was three times higher than that of control participants. The change in serum CC16 concentration was attributed to a transient increase in the lung epithelial permeability, but with no sign of lung function impairment. Ten days after exposure, the CC16 concentration had returned to baseline levels.

When two groups of individuals were compared, a chronic toxic effect on Clara cells was observed in workers inhaling silica-rich dust for an average of 15 months [54]. One group was composed of workers exposed to silica and the other was a control group, matched for age, body mass index and proportion of smokers. After 15 months, the mineworkers showed a significant reduction in serum CC16, even though they did not present any lung function impairment or abnormalities in their chest X-ray. The decrease was reported for both the nonsmokers and the smokers, but an additional and significant effect of tobacco smoking was found. The authors associated this decrease with a reduction in the release of CC16 from the Clara cells probably due to their damage from the toxic action of silica. Pertaining literature suggests that the toxic metabolites of tobacco smoke not only increase the permeability of the lung epithelium, but also cause a progressive destruction of Clara cells [47].

5.1. Studies investigating the effect of air pollution on performance, lung inflammation and injury

Exercise leads to various physiological changes that can aggravate the effects of air pollutants. At resting conditions our breathing is predominantly nasal. This has various advantages which includes not only humidifying and heating the inspired air but also filtering it. Once exercise starts becoming more intense, individuals automatically switch the nasal breathing to oral breathing in an attempt to increase the amount inhaled. Nevertheless avoiding the nasal filtration system potentially enhances the pollutant concentration that reaches the lungs.

With the beginning of exercise, the ventilatory exchange rate (VE) starts to increase and, depending on the exercise intensity and the size of the individual, the VE can be higher than 160 l/min which also leads to an increase in air pollution inhaled. For example, it has been shown that, with the start of an exercise bout, there is an increase in the proportion of ultrafine particles (nanosized particulate matter) inhaled and deposited in the airways but not eliminated [56, 57]. This could be due to impaired nasal mucociliary clearance and reduced cilia beat frequency which can occur with strenuous exercise [58, 59]. This impairment of respiratory defences together with a higher VE and deeper breathing makes the active and athletic population of large cities more vulnerable to the harmful effect of air pollution on health and on performance, especially with long-duration high-intensity exercise. Most of the major sports events (e.g. Summer Olympic Games, Football World Cup) take place within or near large cities, e.g. polluted Olympic Games venues Barcelona 1992; Atlanta 1996; Athens 2004; Beijing 2008; London 2012 [60, 61]. Rio de Janeiro, Brazil's second biggest city (population density of 5346 hab/km^2) and host of the 2016 Olympic Games, also presents high levels of air pollution [5].

Studies that have investigated the deleterious effects of air pollution on performance do indeed report that athletes have an impaired performance [62-64]. This can be further exacerbated depending on other environmental conditions, such as elevated temperature and humidity [65]. This impairment can be attributed not only to an increase in lung inflammation, which can decrease its function, but also to the increase in respiratory symptoms that the athletes experience, including cough, nausea, pain on deep inspiration and wheezing, amongst others. This would lead to a decrease in maximal inspiration volume via neural stimulation of sensory fibers present in the lungs, affecting. In more reactive individuals, the ozone could activate "irritant" receptors leading to contraction of alveolar smooth muscles and as a result changes in respiratory muscle force and mechanic properties of the lungs would occur [66, 67]. Endurance exercise alone has also been shown to decrease lung function because hyperventilation affects the airway smooth muscles [68].

Table 4 presents a summary of studies that have investigated the effect of O_3 air pollution on lung inflammation, injury and function. It is interesting to see the different markers that were analysed, as well as the protocols used. More details of some studies are described below.

Devlin *et al.* [72] analyzed the concentration of a broad range of inflammatory mediators in BAL fluid 1 h after ozone exposure. In this study, volunteers performed intermittent heavy treadmill exercise (66 l min^{-1}) for 2 h in a chamber where the ozone concentration was 0.4 ppm. An increase was observed in mediators of inflammation such as neutrophils, IL-6 and lactate dehydrogenase (LDH), which is an indicator of cell damage. Similarly Holz and colleagues [39] observed a significant increase in neutrophil count and percentage in induced sputum 1 h after participants completed 3 h of light intermittent exercise-14 l min^{-1} m^{-2} of body surface

Study	Subjects	Exercise andOzone levels	Results
Adams & Schelegle, 1983 [69]	Endurance runners	1 h training or competition simulation 0; 0.2; 0.35 ppm	↓ lung funtion at 0.2 and 0.35 ppm ↑ Respiratory symptoms with higher O_3 concentration, impairment in performance
Schelegle & Adams, 1986 [70]	Cyclists	1 h 1 h competitive cycling simulation protocol 0; 0.12; 0.18; and 0.24ppm	↓ lung funtion at 0.18 and 0.24ppm ↑ Respiratory symptoms with higher O_3 concentration, impairment in performance
Brunekreef *et al.*, 1994 [71]	Field study with cyclists	75 min cycling 0.04 – 0.1 ppm + 17,9 ºC	Small ↓ in lung function Correlation between the O3 exposure and the impairement in lung function
Devlin *et al.*, 1996 [72]	Healthy male individuals	2 h heavy intermittent cycling 0.4 ppm	1 h post-exposure = ↑ neutrophil, IL-6 and LDH in BAL
Krishna *et al.*, 1998 [73]	*Healthy individuals	2 h intermittent cycling 0.12 ppm	6 h post-exposure = ↑ neutrophil, IL-8 in BAL No effect on lung function
Blomberg *et al.*, 1999 [38]	*Healthy individuals	2 h intermittent cycling 0.2 ppm	1.5 h post-exposure: no effect on neutrophil count or percentage in BAL, but ↑ in inflammatory mediators ↓ Lung function
Holz *et al.*, 1999 [39]	*Mild asthmatics + nonasthmatics	3 h intermittent cycling 0.12 ppm 0.25 ppm	↑ neutrophil percentage and count in sputum (0.25 ppm O_3) ↑IL-8 in sputum (0.25 ppm O_3) No effect on lung function
Broeckaert *et al.*, 2000 [51]	Field study, trained cyclists	Average 35 km cycling Average 0.076 ppm	Post-exercise = ↑ in serum CC16
Blomberg *et al.*, 2003 [76]	Healthy individuals	2 h intermittent cycling 0.2 ppm	2 h and 4 h post-exposure = ↑ in serum CC16
Lagerkvist *et al.* 2004 [77]	Children (10-11 years of age)	2 h of outdoor exercise 0.059 ppm	No effect on serum CC16 or lung function
Gomes *et al.* 2010 [64] and 2011 [65]	Elite runners	8 km time trial 0.1ppm 31ºC + 70% rh	Immediately post-exercise: ↑ CC16 in NL and no difference on neutrophil counts No effect on lung function Decrease in performance

↑ Increase ↓decrease. *Non-smokers, male and female, the study does not report their physical fitness level.

Table 4. Studies investigating the effect of O_3 after exercise

area-exposed to 0.25 ppm of O_3. Nevertheless, when the participants performed the same exercise bout exposed to a lower O_3 concentration (0.12 ppm), no changes in neutrophils were observed. Furthermore, sputum IL-8 concentration was reported to be elevated only after the 0.25 ppm exposure.

Contrasting some of the previous findings, Blomberg *et al.* [38] were unable to find either mucosal and airway neutrophilia or LDH increase at 1.5 h after a 2 h exposure to 0.2 ppm O_3

in subjects performing intermittent moderate cycling exercise producing an average minute ventilation of 20 l min^{-1} m^{-2} of body surface area. This difference might be explained by the lower exercise and O_3 levels in the latter study which would have as consequence the lowering of the inhaled O_3 dose. Nevertheless, in tissue obtained from bronchial mucosal biopsies, Blomberg *et al.* [38] were able to detect increases in the expression of vascular endothelium P-selectin and ICAM-1 after the ozone exposure. These molecules mediate adhesion and rolling of leukocytes on the vessel walls. Hence, it was suggested that although there was an increase in the expression of vascular adhesion molecules in the vascular endothelium, this had not yet resulted in an increase in neutrophil numbers at the analyzed sites. Stenfors *et al.* [74] using the same study design as the previously-mentioned researchers, demonstrated a significant increase in BAL neutrophil number and percentage 6 h after the exercise trial. In addition, vascular endothelium P-selectin and ICAM-1 were also elevated. This reinforces the importance of these adhesion molecules in the inflammatory response since they recruit inflammatory cells into the airways of healthy individuals.

Gomes and colleagues [64, 65] investigated well trained runners performing an intense exercise bout (8 km time trial) in an environment that, in addition to ozone pollution, was warm and humid. This kind of environment is relevant because the formation of ozone is intensified during the summer when there is a high incidence of sun light. Even though they did not report any changes in lung function, there were signs of lung inflammation and lung injury, the latter observed by an increase in NL CC16 concentration. In addition, there was a positive correlation between lung antioxidant concentrations and performance, that is, the athletes who presented lower concentrations of lung antioxidants were the ones who had a higher impairment in their performance in that extreme environment.

Other studies have also looked into changes in CC16 with exercise associated with ozone pollution. Broeckaert *et al.* [75] investigated 24 non-smoking cyclists, performing a 2 h of moderate intensity cycling during episodes of photochemical smog. The average concentration of ozone was 0.076 ppm. Immediately before and after each ride, the participants provided blood samples and also performed lung function tests. Significant correlations were found between the O_3 concentration and the cyclists' serum levels of CC16 both pre and post-exercise. By contrast, when comparing pre and post rides, no decrease on lung function parameters were found-these are usually impaired by O_3 exposure. Thus, this study showed that short-term exposures to ambient-levels of O_3 induced an early increase in serum CC16 which took place before other manifestations of lung toxicity. However, there was no control group to verify if this increase was due to the exercise, the ozone or a combination of both. The authors suggested that the increase seen in the serum CC16 was due to an increase in the pulmonary epithelium permeability and not to an increase in the production of this protein. As this study was conducted in the field, it is difficult to attribute these results directly to O_3 exposure, as there may have been other pollutants that could also have influenced the epithelial leakage. In addition, the levels of serum CC16 pre-ride were also correlated with the levels of ambient O_3, indicating that the cyclists initiated the exercise with an increased lung epithelium permeability.

Blomberg *et al.* [76] conducted a lab study where 22 subjects performed 2 h of moderate intermittent exercise. They were exposed to two different environment conditions: 0.2 ppm of O_3 and filtered air. The participants' lung function was assessed and peripheral blood samples were obtained 2 h pre, immediately pre, immediately post, 2 and 4 h post-exercise. Significant decreases in the lung function parameters, FEV_1 and FVC, were observed immediately post O_3 exposure. However, at 2 and 4 h post-exercise this decrease was no longer observed. Moreover, a significant increase in CC16 serum levels was seen around 2 and 4 h post O_3 exposure. No relationship was noted between CC16 and lung function at any of the analyzed points. Serum CC16 concentrations were shown to have returned to baseline 18 h post-exposure. Other epithelial permeability markers, albumin and total protein concentration, which were also assessed, did not show a significant increase. The data from this study supports the theory that serum CC16 is a more sensitive marker of altered lung epithelial permeability when compared to traditional markers.

Contrary to the above-mentioned studies, Lagerkvist *et al.* [77] did not find any significant changes in serum levels of CC16 in children (10-11 years of age). They performed 2 h of outdoor exercise, where the maximal O_3 value reached 0.059 ppm. Blood samples and lung function performance were analyzed pre and post-exercise. Yet no decrease in lung function or changes in CC16 were observed. In relation to CC16 concentration, the authors reported that children who regularly visited chlorinated indoor swimming pools presented significantly lower levels of serum CC16 both before and after the outdoor exercise when compared to the non-swimming children. In this study, it is important to observe that the maximum level of O_3 reported is lower than in the previous studies discussed above. Furthermore, the authors mentioned that the children performed light exercise; though, they did not report the type of exercise nor how the exercise intensity was controlled. More investigation is needed to establish the effect of ozone and exercise on airway permeability of different populations, as there are still contradictions in the literature using CC16 as a marker of lung injury.

Acute exposure to ozone, as investigated in the studies above, is very relevant and can also be related to some real-life situations when cities experience intense pollution episodes or when individuals travel to more polluted areas. Nevertheless, chronic exposure to air pollution also needs further investigation. Unfortunately, several challenges are present for the development of research on chronic exposure to air pollution on a human exercising population. Christian *et al.* [53] showed an attenuation of the inflammatory response in BAL after four consecutive days of exposure to ozone. Nevertheless, it seems that, although neutrophil recruitment and IL-6 concentration in the respiratory tract is attenuated with multiday short-term exposures, airway epithelial injury may continue to occur. The data from Jörres *et al.* [44] support the previous finding, with them additionally reporting that, after four consecutive exposures, an increase in airway mucosa inflammation as well as the neutrophil count was observed in bronchial mucosal biopsies. These data, thus, demonstrate that airway inflammation persists despite the attenuation of some inflammatory markers in BAL. It is important to point out that such persistent injury could lead to airway remodeling, which has been observed in several animal studies, but needs further investigation in humans [53].

Using a different technique, sputum induction, to assess airway inflammation, Ratto *et al.* [45] found an increase in the percentage of neutrophils after 4 h of 0.2 ppm O_3 exposure during 4 consecutive days. This finding is in contrast to the afore-mentioned studies using BAL where it was observed an attenuation of the inflammatory response. Nevertheless, the increased recruitment of neutrophils to proximal airway tissue, showed by the analysis of induced sputum, was consistent with the examination of endobronchial biopsies samples taken by Jörres *et al.* [44]. Once more, it shows that different techniques sample different airway compartments producing differing results. In addition, the exposure and exercise protocol is also essential for the outcome of the inflammatory process. An important additional factor that appears to affect results in these studies is individual responsiveness due to differences in ozone sensitivity of individuals [39, 78].

6. Air pollution, exercise and antioxidant supplementation

The respiratory tract lining fluid is the first barrier encountered by inspired gases and, therefore, it has a network of antioxidants, such as ascorbic acid, GSH, α-tocopherol and uric acid to provide protection against oxidative stress [42, 78, 79]. For this reason, antioxidant supplementation has been suggested as a benefit for people exercising in an air-polluted environment. The rationale behind such hypothesis is that increasing the availability of antioxidants in the respiratory-tract lining fluid will provide additional sacrificial substrates for the oxidant-be it PM, O_3 or any other oxidant gas. These additional sacrificial substrates will, in turn, decrease oxidation reactions occurring within this fluid and within the under-lining epithelial cells. In addition, an excess in antioxidants concentration might also confer protection by neutralizing free radical species, derived from these initial reactions or inflammatory cells [26, 78]. As a result, the toxicity of the pollutant would be decreased limiting the inflammation response of the cells from the epithelium tract [80], consequently, lung injury would be minimized and lung function would be maintained.

Some studies have investigated this proposed benefit of increasing antioxidant availability in individuals exposed to ozone-pollution by supplementing the participants with a mix of antioxidants, mostly vitamins C and E. These two antioxidants are present in the RTLF, they both have strong antioxidant properties and together have been shown to present a synergistic effect in the protection against oxidative stress [78, 81]. Vitamin E is the major lipophilic antioxidant in human tissues, whether in the airways or otherwise; and vitamin C has been linked to maintenance of lung health, as for example, by improving lung function, having a positive effect on exercise-induced bronchoconstriction in asthmatic individuals and decreasing the adverse respiratory symptoms experienced during exercise [82-84]. As will be further elucidated, supplementation with these two vitamins has been shown to provide some protection in humans exposed to ozone-pollution [35, 85-88]. Little is known in relation to the benefits of antioxidants when it comes to exposure to other kinds of air pollutants other than O_3. Nevertheless, the benefits would be expected to be similar for all the oxidant air pollutants.

Romieu *et al.* [85] have shown the existence of some protective effect when participants are supplemented with a mix of antioxidants. These researchers conducted a field study in which

34 workers (shoe-cleaners), who were constantly exposed to pollution (Mexico City), participated in a double blind supplementation/placebo crossover design study. The supplementation consisted of a mix of different antioxidants (650 mg vitamin C+100 IU vitamin E+15 mg b-carotene) ingested during a 10-week period. The washout period was 2 weeks. The average daily ozone concentration was 0.07 ppm, and on 55% of the days the concentration exceeded the Mexican standard of 0.11 ppm. As reported, antioxidant supplementation resulted in a protective effect on the lung function against the ozone exposure. The authors, however, do mention that individuals who consumed antioxidants first presented less lung function impairment after consuming placebo than subjects that initially ingested placebo. The authors attributed this result to the short washout period, especially in relation to vitamin E, which accumulates in the tissues; but they did not investigate this issue. Field studies, such as this one, have some limitations, as for instance, the interference of other pollutants and the change in concentration of the analyzed pollutant throughout the long period in which the study was conducted. In addition, the participants of this study were not exercising while being exposed to the pollution.

Two subsequent field studies, conducted with amateur and recreational cyclists [86, 87], reached similar results in relation to antioxidant supplementation providing some protection against the acute effects of ozone on lung function. Grievink *et al.* [86] observed two groups of cyclists, during a 3-month period. One group was supplemented with vitamin C (650 mg day^{-1}), vitamin E (100 IU day^{-1}) and β-carotene (15 mg day^{-1}); while the other group ingested placebo. This study was conducted during the summer months, and the lung function of the cyclists was measured before and after training or competition on 4 to 14 occasions. Of note, the supplementation started 1 week before the first measurement and was maintained during the study period, and this could have influenced the result as the participants were not all tested on the same occasions. The mean temperature throughout the study period was 23°C and the ozone concentration averaged 0.05 ppm. In the subsequent study by these researchers [87], the same protocol was followed in relation to the exercise and measurements during the summer; however, the supplementation protocol varied slightly (3 months of daily vitamin C 500 mg and vitamin E 150 IU). In this later study, even though it was reported that the supplementation was able to partly counteract the decreases of lung function, the authors also mentioned that, when participants who had not complied fully with the supplementation were excluded from the analysis, the effects of ozone on lung function were no longer observed. The average temperature and ozone concentration in this study were lower than in the previous study: 17°C and 0.04 ppm respectively. Both studies presented some disadvantages. Firstly, they analysed two different groups of individuals, making comparison challenging as the effects of ozone have been shown to vary a lot from one individual to another. Secondly, the placebo group and the vitamin group were not balanced in relation to individuals presenting respiratory allergies or asthma. In addition, in the latter study [87], the placebo group, acting as the control, was not taking any pills, therefore, it was not blinded. Thirdly, some individuals in the supplemented group were already taking antioxidants prior to the start of the study. Lastly, it was reported that the adjustment for environmental temperature as a possible confounder was difficult due to the high correlation with ozone. All in all, it is important to view these results with caution because this array of uncontrolled variables could have influenced the outcome.

In the study of Samet *et al.* [35], participants were divided into two groups and all underwent a 1-week period of vitamin C-restricted diet. After this, one of the groups received supplementation (250 mg vitamin C+50 IU vitamin E+12 oz of carrot and tomato juice), while the other group received placebo and continued on the restricted diet. The supplementation period consisted of a 2-week period after which the subjects underwent a 2 h low-intensity exercise protocol in a high ozone-polluted chamber (0.4 ppm). After exposure, the subjects completed a respiratory symptom questionnaire, performed lung function tests and underwent a bronchoalveolar lavage. There were no differences between the supplemented group and the placebo group in respect to answers given in the respiratory symptom questionnaire. This suggests that dietary antioxidants do not minimize the perceived harmful effects of ozone. In addition, there were no differences in neutrophil counts or other inflammatory markers in the bronchoalveolar lavage fluid. Nevertheless, the authors did report attenuation in lung function impairment in relation to the subjects who ingested the antioxidant mixture.

Contrary to this finding, Mudway *et al.* (89) did not report any changes in lung function when they conducted a double-blind crossover study. The supplementation (500 mg vitamin C+150 IU vitamin E daily) period in this study was smaller than most supplementation protocols: just 1 week, with a 2-week washout period. The exposure protocol consisted of 2 h of intermittent cycling in a chamber with 0.2 ppm of ozone. Besides the lack of changes in lung function, there were no differences in airway inflammation, which was assessed 6 h post-exposure. It is important to point out that, after the supplementation protocol, the subjects did present an increased concentration of plasma ascorbic acid and α-tocopherol. This increased concentration, however, was not observed in the respiratory airways when it was accessed 6 h after the ozone exposure. Nevertheless, the authors did report movement of α-tocopherol from the plasma into the RTLF following the ozone challenge.

In a 2011 study, Gomes et al [90] reported that there was a positive effect of a 2-week supplementation period of vitamin E and vitamin C on the pre-exercise levels of the total antioxidant concentration in the RTLF. In addition, after the 8 km time trial run the participants, when on the vitamins, presented decreased lung injury (higher CC16 levels in both the plasma and NL) compared to when they took the placebos. Participants also ran on average 49sec faster when taking the vitamins. The environment where the exercise took place had, besides the ozone pollution (0.1ppm), also heat and humidity. This study was also conducted in a double-blinded randomized and crossover way, which minimizes biases. A summary of the studies presented above is provided in Table 5.

The inconclusiveness of the literature can possibly be attributed to divergences in the methodologies used in the research, such as different supplementation protocols, exercise modes and participants' fitness levels. Additionally, only one study looked at the effect of antioxidant supplementation on performance in a polluted environment, with more information being necessary in relation to the antioxidant and inflammatory response. Due to the high antioxidant consumption by the physically active community and by a large portion of the general

Study	Subjects	Design	Supplement	Exercise and ozone levels	Results
Romieu *et al*., 1998 [85]	Shoe-cleaners	Field study Crossover (n=34)	10 wks: vit C 650 mg + vit E 100 IU + b-carotene + 15 mg daily	Daily work Average of 0.07 ppm O_3	Attenuation of lung function impairment with supplementation
Grievink *et al*., 1998 [86]	Amateur and recreational cyclists	Field study Placebo (n =18) Supplemented (n=20)	Started 1 wk before 1st measurement, total of 3 months: vit C 650mg + vit E 100 IU and b-carotene 15mg daily	Training sessions Average of 0.05 ppm O_3	Supplementation provided some protection on lung function
Grievink *et al*., 1999 [87]	Amateur cyclists	Field study Placebo (n =9) Supplemented (n=11)	Started 1 wk before first measurement, total of 3 months: vit C 500 mg + vit E 150 IU daily	Training sessions and competitive races Average of 0.04 ppm O3	No effect on lung function
Samet *et al*., 2001 [35]	Male and female, physical fitness not specified	Placebo (n =16) Supplemented (n=15)	Placebo: 3 wks vitamin restriction Supplemented: 1 wk vitamin restriction + 2 weeks of 250 mg vitamin C + vitamin E 50 IU + 12 oz of carrot and tomato juice daily	2 h low-intensity intermittent exercise on treadmill or cycling 0.4 ppm O_3	Attenuation of lung function decrements with supplementation No differences in respiratory symptoms or lung inflammation
Mudway *et al*., 2006 [89]	Male and female, physical fitness not specified	Crossover (n=14)	1 week: vit C 500mg + vit E 150 IU daily	2 h intermittent cycling 0.2 ppm O_3	No effect on lung function No effect on lung inflammation
Gomes et al. 2011 [90]	Male elite runners	Crossover (n=10)	2 weeks: vit C 500mg + vit E 100 IU daily	8km time trial run	Attenuation of lung injury with supplementation 49 sec improvement in performance

Table 5. Studies investigating vitamin C and E supplementation in ozone exposure

population, this is an important topic for research, particularly when coupled with the fact that large urbanized areas might provide an additional reason, in the form of air pollutants, to increase the antioxidant intake.

7. Chapter summary

The main points of this chapter are:

- Air pollution can be found both indoor and outdoor. Sources of air pollution are mainly found in urban areas linked to human activities, such as power plants, and locations where there are high concentration of vehicles and burning of fossil fuel. Some pollutants are also generated by natural processes.
- Air pollutants can be found in different forms and sizes and they can exist as solid particles, liquid molecules or gases. Some examples include: Ozone, particulate matter, carbon monoxide, and nitrogen dioxide.
- High levels of air pollutants have been shown to cause and exacerbate various pulmonary and cardiovascular diseases, as well as increase mortality. Low birth weight and baby development have also been shown to occur in areas with high levels of air pollution.
- The active population that exercise and compete outdoors are a susceptible group. This is the case because exercise leads to an increase in the amount and depth of air that is inhaled, which results in higher doses of air pollutants reaching deeper places in the lungs. This also facilitates the passage of the smaller sized PM into the systemic circulation.
- Some air pollutants can trigger an oxidative stress process in the lungs which can lead to cell death, inflammation, injury and loss of function.
- Antioxidants are sacrificial molecules that promptly react with free radicals and reactive species neutralizing them. There is a wide range of antioxidants in body fluids, tissues and organs, working synergistically in a network
- CC16 is a small-sized protein which changes in concentrations can indicate lung injury and toxicity. It can be measured in the upper and lower respiratory tract, as well as in the blood.
- Performance could be affected when individuals exercise in an ozone polluted environment. This, however, depends on the exercise type, intensity, duration, individual susceptibility and other environmental factors, such as heat and humidity.
- Although more studies are necessary, antioxidant supplementation might help to mitigate the adverse effect of ozone pollution on health and performance.

Author details

Elisa Couto Gomes and Geraint Florida-James*

*Address all correspondence to: g.florida-james@napier.ac.uk

School of Life, Sport and Social Sciences, Edinburgh Napier University, United Kingdom

References

[1] Brook RD, Franklin B, Cascio W, Hong Y, Howard G, Lipsett M, et al. Air pollution and cardiovascular disease: a statement for healthcare professionals from the Expert Panel on Population and Prevention Science of the American Heart Association. *Circulation* 2004; 109: 2655–2671.

[2] Cohen AJ, Anderson HR, Ostro B, Pandey KD, Krzyzanowski M, Kunzli N, et al. Mortality impacts of urban air pollution. In: Ezzati M, Lopez AD, Rodgers A, Murray CJL (eds) *Comparative quantifcation of health risks:global and regional burden of disease attributable to selected major risk factors*. Geneva, World Health Organization; 2004. p1353–1434.

[3] Bell ML, Davis DL, Gouveia N, Borja-Aburto VH, Cifuentes LA. The avoidable health effects of air pollution in three Latin American cities: Santiago, Sao Paulo, and Mexico City. *Environmental Research* 2006; 100: 431-440.

[4] Lewtas J. Air pollution combustion emissions: characterization of causative agents and mechanisms associated with cancer, reproductive, and cardiovascular effects. *Mutation Research* 2007; 636 (1-3): 95-133.

[5] Romieu I, Gouveia N, Cifuentes LA, de Leon AP, Junger W, Vera J et al. (2012). Multicity study of air pollution and mortality in Latin America (the ESCALA study). *Respiratory Report Health Effects Institute* 2012; 171: 5-86.

[6] Brunekreef B, Holgatek ST. Air pollution and health. *The Lancet* 2002; 360: 1233-1242.

[7] Katsouyanni K. Ambient air pollution and health. *British Medical Bulletin* 2003; 68: 143-156.

[8] Brauer M, Lencar C, Tamburic L, Koehoorn M, Demers P, Karr C. A cohort study of traffic-related air pollution impacts on birth outcomes. *Environmental Health Perspectives* 2008; 116(5):680-686.

[9] Morello-Frosch R, Jesdale BM, Sadd JL, Pastor M. Ambient air pollution exposure and full-term birth weight in California. *Environmental Health: a global acess science source* 2010; 9:44.

[10] Savitz DA, Bobb JF, Carr JL, Clougherty JE, Dominici F, Elston B, et al. Ambient Fine Particulate Matter, Nitrogen Dioxide, and Term Birth Weight in New York, New York. *American Journal of Epidemiology* 2013; [Epub ahead of print] DOI: 10.1093/aje/kwt268 (accessed 05 December 2012).

[11] Le TG, Ngo L, Mehta S, Do VD, Thach TQ, Vu XD, et al. Effects of short-term exposure to air pollution on hospital admissions of young children for acute lower respiratory infections in Ho Chi Minh City, Vietnam. *Research Report Health Effects Institute* 2012; 169: 5-83.

[12] Yap et alYap PS, Gilbreath S, Garcia C, Jareen N, Goodrich B. The influence of socioeconomic markers on the association between fine particulate matter and hospital admissions for respiratory conditions among children. *American Journal of Public Health* 2013; 103(4):695-702.

[13] Stedman JR. The predicted number of air pollution related deaths in the UK during the August 2003 heatwave. *Atmospheric Environment* 2004; 38: 1087-1090.

[14] Bates DV. Ambient ozone and mortality. *Epidemiology* 2005; 16 (4): 427-429.

[15] Krzyzanowski M, Cohen A. Update of WHO air quality guidelines. Air Quality and Atmosphere Health 2008; 1: 7-13.

[16] Global estimates of burden of disease caused by the environmental and occupational risks http://www.who.int/quantifying_ehimpacts/global/urbair/en/index.html 2007 (accessed 07 November 2012).

[17] An X, Zhu T, Wang Z, Li C, Wang Y. A modeling analysis of a heavy air pollution episode occurred in Beijing. Atmosmospheric Chemistry and Physics Discussion 2006; 6: 8215–8240.

[18] Menzies D, Nair A, Williamson PA, Schembri S, Al-Khairalla MZ, Barnes M, et al. Respiratory symptoms, pulmonary function, and markers of inflammation among bar workers before and after a legislative ban on smoking in public places. JAMA 2006; 296 (14): 1742–8.

[19] Ayres JG, Semple S, MacCalman L, Dempsey S, Hilton S, Hurley JF, et al. Bar workers' health and environmental tobacco smoke exposure (BHETSE): symptomatic improvement in bar staff following smoke-free legislation in Scotland. *Occupational and Environmental Medicine* 2009; 66: 339-346.

[20] Kent BD, Sulaiman I, Nicholson TT, Lane SJ, Moloney ED. Acute pulmonary admissions following implementation of a national workplace smoking ban. *Chest* 2012; 142(3): 673-679.

[21] Millett C, Lee JT, Laverty AA, Glantz SA, Majeed A. Hospital admissions for childhood asthma after smoke-free legislation in England. *Pediatrics* 2013; 131(2): e495-501.

[22] Sims M, Maxwell R, Gilmore A. Short-term impact of the smoke-free legislation in England on emergency hospital admissions for asthma among adults: a population-based study. *Thorax* 2013; 68(7): 619-24.

[23] Cronin EM, Kearney PM, Kearney PP, Sullivan P, Perry IJ; Coronary Heart Attack Ireland Registry (CHAIR) Working Group. Impact of a national smoking ban on hospital admission for acute coronary syndromes: a longitudinal study. *Clinical Cardiology* 2012; 35(4): 205-209.

[24] Herman PM, Walsh ME. Hospital admissions for acute myocardial infarction, angina, stroke, and asthma after implementation of Arizona's comprehensive statewide smoking ban. *American Journal of Public Health* 2011; 101(3): 491-496.

[25] Pryor WA. Mechanisms of radical formation from reactions of ozone with target molecules in the lung. *Free Radical Biology & Medicine* 1994; 17 (5): 451-465.

[26] Pryor WA, Squadrito GL, Friedman M. The cascade mechanism to explain ozone toxicity: the role of lipid ozonation products. *Free Radical Biology and Medicine* 1995, 19, 935-941.

[27] Corradi M, Alinovi R, Goldoni M, Vettori M, Folesani G, Mozzoni P, et al. Biomarkers of oxidative stress after controlled human exposure to ozone. *Toxicology Letters* 2002; 134: 219-225.

[28] Radák Z. *Free Radicals in Exercise and Aging*. Champaign, IL: Human Kinetics; 2000.

[29] Powers SK, DeRuisseau KC, Quindry J, Hamilton KL. Dietary antioxidants and exercise. *Journal of Sports Science* 2004; 22: 81-94.

[30] Halliwell B, Gutteridge, JMC. *Free Radicals in Biology and Medicine*. 3rd ed. New York: Oxford University Press; 2007.

[31] Kuby J (1997). *Immunology*. 3rd ed. New York: W.H. Freeman and Company; 1997.

[32] Sen CK. Antioxidant and redox regulation of cellular signaling: introduction. *Medicine & Science in Sports & Exercise* 2001; 33(3): 368–370.

[33] Cantin AM, North SL, Hubbard RC, Crystal RG. Normal alveolar epithelial lining fluid contains high levels of glutathione. *Journal of Applied Physiology* 1987 ; 63(1): 152-157.

[34] Peden DB, Hohman R, Brown ME, Mason RT, Berkebile C, Fales H M, et al. Uric acid is a major antioxidant in human nasal airway secretions. *Proceedings of the National Academy of Science USA* 1990; 87: 7638-7642.

[35] Samet JM, Hatch GE, Horstman D, Steck-Scott S, Arab L, Bromberg PA, et al. Effect of Antioxidant Supplementation on Ozone-Induced Lung Injury in Human Subjects. *American Journal of Respiratory and Critical Care Medicine* 2001; 164: 819-825.

[36] Housley DG, Mudway I, Kelly FJ, Eccles R, Richards RJ. Depletion of urate in human nasal lavage following in vitro ozone exposure. *International Journal of Biochemistry and Cellular Biology* 1995; 27: 1153-1159.

[37] Mudway SI, Krishna MT, Frew AJ, MacLeod D, Sandstrom T, Holgate ST, et al. Comprised concentrations of ascorbate in fluid lining the respiratory tract in human subjects after exposure to ozone. *Occupational and Environmental Medicine* 1999; 56: 473-481.

[38] Blomberg A, Mudway IS, Nordenhäll C, Hedenström H, Kelly FJ, Frew AJ, et al. Ozone-induced lung function decrements do not correlate with early airway inflammatory or antioxidant responses. *European Respiratory Journal* 1999; 13: 1418-1428.

[39] Holz O, Jörres RA, Timm P, Mücke M, Richter K, Koschyk S, et al. Ozone-induced inflammatory changes differ between individuals and are reproducible. *American Journal of Respiratory and Critical Care Medicine* 1999; 159: 776-784.

[40] Steensberg A, van Hall G, Osada T, Sacchetti M, Saltin B, Pedersen BK. Production of interleukin-6 in contracting human skeletal muscles can account for the exercise-induced increase in plasma interleukin-6. *Journal of Physiology* 2000, 529.1: 237-242.

[41] Febbraio MA, Pedersen BK. Muscle-derived interleukin-6: mechanisms for activation and possible biological roles. *The FASEB Journal* 2002; 16: 1335-1347.

[42] Mudway IS, Blomberg A, Frew AJ, Holgate ST, Sandström T, Kelly FJ. Antioxidant consumption and repletion kinetics in nasal lavage fluid following exposure of healthy human volunteers to ozone. *European Respiratory Journal* 1999; 13: 1429-1438.

[43] Blomberg A. Airway inflammatory and antioxidant responses to oxidative and particulate air pollutants – experimental exposure studies in humans. *Clinical and Experimental Allergy* 2000; 30: 310-317.

[44] Jörres RA, Holz O, Zachgo W, Timm P, Koscyk S, Müller B, et al. The effect of repeated ozone exposures on inflammatory markers in bronchoalveolar lavage fluid and mucosal biopsies. *American Journal of Respiratory and Critical Care Medicine* 2000; 161: 1855-1861.

[45] Ratto J, Wong H, Liu J, Fahy J, Boushey H, Solomon C, et al. Effects of multiday exposure to ozone on airway inflammation as determined using sputum induction. *Environmental Health Perspectives* 2006; 114: 209-212.

[46] Hermans C, Bernard A. Lung epithelium-specific proteins. Characteristics and potential applications as markers (State of art). *American Journal of Respiratory and Critical Care Medicine* 1999; 159: 646-678.

[47] Robin M, Dong P, Hermans C, Bernard A, Bersten AD, Doyle IR. Serum levels of CC16, SP-A and SP-B reflect tobacco-smoke exposure in asymptomatic subjects. *European Respiratory Journal* 2002; 20: 1152-1161.

[48] Broeckaert F, Bernard A. Clara cell secretory protein (CC16): characteristics and perspectives as lung peripheral biomarker. *Clinical & Experimental Allergy* 2000; 30: 469-475.

[49] Helleday R, Segerstedt B, Forsberg B, Mudway I, Nordberg G, Bernard A, Blomberg A. Exploring the time dependence of serum clara cell protein as a biomarker of pulmonary injury in humans. *Chest* 2006; 130: 672-675.

[50] Hermans C, Knoops B, Wiedig M, Arsalene K, Toubeau G, Falmagne P, Bernard A. Clara cell protein as a marker of clara cell damage and bronchoalveolar blood barrier permeability. *European Respiratory Journal* 1999; 13: 1014-1021.

[51] Broeckaert F, Arsalene K, Hermans C, Bergamaschi E, Brustolin A, Muff A.. Serum clara cell protein: a sensitive biomarker of increased lung epithelium permeability caused by ambient ozone. *Environmental health Perspectives* 2000; 108: 533-537.

[52] Gioldassi XM, Papadimitriou H, Mikraki V, Karamanos NK. Clara cell secretory protein: determination of serum levels by na enzyme immunoassay and its importance as an indicator of bronchial asthma in children. *Journal of Pharmaceutical and Biomedical Analysis* 2003; 34(4): 823-826.

[53] Christian DL, Chen LL, Scannel CH, Ferrando RE, Welch BS, Balmes JR. Ozone-induced inflammation is attenuated with multiday exposure. *American Journal of Respiratory and Critical Care Medicine* 1998; 158: 532-537.

[54] Bernard A, Gonzales-Lorenzo JM, Siles E, Trujillano G, Lawerys R. Early decrease of serum Clara cell protein in silica-exposed workers. *European Respiratory Journal* 1994; 7: 1932-1937.

[55] Bernard A, Hermans C, Van Houte G. Transient increase of Clara cell protein (CC16) after exposure to smoke. *Occupational and Environmental Medicine* 1997; 54: 63-65.

[56] Chalupa DC, Morrow PE, Oberdorster G, Utell MJ, Frampton MW. Ultrafine particle deposition in subjects with asthma. *Environmental Health Perspectives* 2004;112(8): 879-82.

[57] Daigle CC, Chalupa DC, Gibb FR, Morrow PE, Oberdorster G, Utell MJ et al. Ultrafine particledeposition in humans during rest and exercise. *Inhalation Toxicology* 2003;15(6): 539-52.

[58] Muns G, Singer P, Wolf F, Rubinstein I. Impaired nasal mucociliary clearance in long-distance runners. *International Journal of Sports Medicine* 1995;16(4):209-13.

[59] Salzano FA, Manola M, Tricarico D, Precone D, Motta G. [Mucociliary clearance after aerobic exertion in athletes]. Acta Otorhinolaryngologica Italica. 2000; 20(3):171-6.

[60] Peiser B, Reilley T. Environmental factors in the summer Olympics in historical perspective. *Journal of Sports Sciences* 2004; 22: 981-1002.

[61] Streets DG, Fu JS, Jang CJ, Hao HK, Tang X, Zhang Y, et al. Air quality during the 2008 Beijing Olympic Games. *Atmospheric Environment* 2007; 41: 480-492.

[62] Gibbons SI, Adams WC. Combined effects of ozone exposure and ambient heat on exercising females. *Journal of Applied Physiology: Respiratory Environment and Exercise Physiology* 1984; 57: 450-456.

[63] Gong HJ, Bradley PW, Simmons MS, Tashkin DP. Impaired exercise performance and pulmonary function in elite cyclists during low-level ozone exposure in a hot environment. *American Review of Respiratory Disease* 1986; 134: 726-733.

[64] Gomes EC, Stone V, Florida-James G. Investigating performance and lung function in a hot, humid and ozone-polluted environment. *European Journal of Applied Physiology* 2010; 110(1): 199-205.

[65] Gomes EC, Stone V, Florida-James G. Impact of heat and pollution on oxidative stress and CC16 secretion after 8 km run. *European Journal of Applied Physiology* 2011; 111(9): 2089-2097.

[66] Passannante A, Hazucha MJ, Bromberg PA, Seal E, Folisbee L, Koch G. Nocioceptive mechanisms modulate ozone-induced human lung function decrements. *Journal of Applied Physiology* 1998; 85(5): 1863-1870.

[67] Hazucha MJ, Bates DV, Bromberg PA. Mechanism of action of ozone on the human lung. *Journal of Applied Physiology* 1989; 67 (4): 1535-1541.

[68] Scichilone N, Morice G, Marchese R, Bonanno A, Profita M, Togias A, Bonsignore MR. Reduced airway responsiveness in nonelite runners. *Medicine & science in Sport & Exercise* 2005; 37 (12): 2019-2025.

[69] Adams WC, Schelegle SE. Ozone and high ventilation effects on pulmonary function and endurance performance. *Journal of Applied Physiology: Respiratory, Environmental and Exercise Physiology* 1983; 55: 805-812.

[70] Schelegle ES, Adams WC. Reduced exercise time in competitive simulations consequent to low level ozone exposure. *Medicine & science in Sport & Exercise* 1986; 18: 408-414.

[71] Brunekreef B, Hoek G, Breugelmans O, Leentvaar M. Respiratory effects of low-level photochemical air pollution in amateur cyclists. *American Journal of Respiratory and Critical Care Medicine* 1994; 150: 962-966.

[72] Devlin RB, McDonnel WF, Becker S, Madden MC, McGee MP, Perez R, et al. Time-dependent changes of inflammatory mediators in the lungs of humans exposed to 0.4 ppm ozone for 2 hr: a comparison of mediators found in the bronchoalveolar lavage fluid 1 and 18 hs after exposure. *Toxicology and Applied Pharmacology* 1996; 138: 176-185.

[73] Krishna MT, Madden J, Teran LM, Biscione GL, Lau LC, Withers NJ, et al. Effects of 0.2 ppm ozone on biomarkers of inflammation in bronchoalveolar lavage fluid and bronchial mucosa of healthy subjects. *European Respiratory Journal* 1998; 11: 1294-1300.

[74] Stenfors N, Pourazar J, Blomberg A, Krishna MT, Mudway I, Helleday R, et al. Effect of ozone on bronchial mucosal inflammation in asthmatic and healthy subjects. *Respiratory Medicine* 2002; 96: 352-358.

[75] Broeckaert F, Clippe A, Knoops B, Hermans C, Bernard A. The impact Clara cell secretory protein (CC16): features as a peripheral lung biomarker. *Annals New York Academy of Science* 2000; 923: 68-77.

[76] Blomberg A, Mudway I, Svensson M, Hagenbjörk-Gustafssonz A, Thomassonz L, Helleday R, et al. Clara cell protein as a biomarker for ozone-induced lung injury in humans. *European Respiratory Journal* 2003; 22: 883-888.

[77] Lagerkvist BJ, Bernard A, Blomberg A, bergstrom E, Forsberg B, Holmstrom K, et al. Pulmonary epithelial integrity in children: relationship to ambient ozone exposure and swimming pool attendance. *Environmental Health Perspectives* 2004; 112: 1768-1771.;

[78] Mudway IS, Stenfors N, Blomberg A, Helleday R, Dunster C, Marklund SL, et al. Differences in basal airway antioxidant concentrations are not predictive of individual responsiveness to ozone: a comparison of healthy and mild asthmatic subjects. *Free Radical Biology and Medicine* 2001, 31(8), 962-974.

[79] Van Der Vliet A, O'Neil CA, Cross CE, Koostra JM, Volz WG, Halliwell B, et al. Determination of low-molecular-mass antioxidant concentrations in human respiratory tract lining fluids. *American Journal of Physiology (Lung Cellular and Molecular Physiology)* 1999; 276: L289-296.

[80] Kelly FJ. Dietary antioxidants and environmental stress. *Proceedings of the Nutrition Society* 2004; 63: 579–585.

[81] Rietjens IMCM, Boersma MG, Haan L, Spenkelink B, Awad HM, Cnubben NHP, et al. The pro-oxidant chemistry of the natural antioxidants vitamin C, vitamin E, carotenoids and flavonoids. *Environmental Toxicology and Pharmacology* 2002; 11: 321-333.

[82] Cross CE, Vasu VT, Lim Y, Gohil K. Combating oxidative stress at respiratory biosurfaces: challenges yet to be resolved, a commentary on "Vitamin supplementation does not protect against symptoms in ozone-responsive subjects". *Free Radical Biology and Medicine* 2006; 40: 1693-1697.

[83] Romieu I, Varraso R, Avenel V, Leynaert B, Kauffmann F, Clavel-Chapelo F. Fruit and vegetable intakes and asthma in the E3N study. *Thorax* 2006; 61: 209-215.

[84] Teckenburg SL, Mickleborough TD, Fly AD, Bai Y, Stager JM. Ascorbic acid supplementation attenuates exercise-induced bronchoconstriction in patients with asthma. *Respiratory Medicine* 2007; 101: 1770-1778.

[85] Romieu I, Meneses F, Ramirez M, Ruiz S, Padilla RP, Sienra JJ, et al. Antioxidant Supplementation and Respiratory Functions among Workers Exposed to *High Levels of Ozone. American Journal of Respiratory and Critical Care Medicine* 1998; 158: 226-232.

[86] Grievink L, Jansen SM, Veer PVT, Brunekreef B. Acute effects of ozone on pulmonary function of cyclists receiving antioxidant supplements. *Occupational and Environmental Medicine* 1998; *55*: 13-17.

[87] Grievink L, Zijlstra AG, Ke X, Brunekreef B. Double-Blind Intervention Trial on Modulation of Ozone Effects on Pulmonary Function by Antioxidant Supplements. *American Journal of Epidemiology* 1999, 149 (4), 306-314.

[88] Sienra-Monge JJ, Ramirez-Aguilar M, Moreno-Macias H, Reyez-Ruiz NI, Del Rio-Navarro BE, Hatch G, et al. Antioxidant supplementation and nasal inflammatory responses among young asthmatics exposed to high levels of ozone. *Clinical and Experimental Immunology* 2004; 138: 317-322.

[89] Mudway IS, Behdig AF, Helleday R, Pourazar J, Frew AJ, Kelly FJ, Blomberg A. Vitamin supplementation does not protect against symptoms in ozone-responsive subjects. *Free Radical Biology and Medicine* 2006; 40, 1702-1712.

[90] Gomes EC, Allgrove JE, Florida-James G, Stone V. Effect of Vitamin Supplementation on Lung Injury and Running Performance in a Hot, Humid and Ozone Polluted Environment. Scandinavian Journal of Medicine & Science in Sports 2011; 21(6): e452-460.

Chapter 2

Macrophage Polarization in Lung Biology and Diseases

Leema George, Swapna Upadhyay,
Koustav Ganguly and Tobias Stoeger

Additional information is available at the end of the chapter

http://dx.doi.org/10.5772/57567

1. Introduction

Lung is a major site of continuous immune reactions as it encounters various foreign particles and antigens entering the respiratory system. It is the main internal organ constantly exposed to the external environment that contains an array of microbes and particulate matter. Typically an adult exchanges 4.2 liters of air per minute amounting to almost 6000 liters per day [1In fact ventilation and respiration generates an environment where both inflammatory and anti-inflammatory response takes place continuously. However, a delicate balance is maintained between eliciting an immune response followed by resolution and repression of further immune reactions. Uncontrolled responses may result in injury or collateral damage to the lung whereas a subdued immune reaction may lead to unchecked infection. Hence, an efficient inflammatory reaction followed by precisely controlled resolution and fine-tuned remodeling process has evolved to minimize the effects of such challenges. The immune system of the lung is well developed to encounter this continuous challenge and disparate demands. Both innate and adaptive immune responses contribute to the surveillance of overall immune function in the lung. The respective immunological effector cells, T-lymphocytes, mast cells, dendritic cells (DCs) and macrophages are present within the lung interstitium, as early as from the pseudoglandular stage of development [2].

Macrophages are strategically distributed all over the body, present virtually in all tissues. They represent an important part of the immune system as tissue resident cells. Macrophages can differentiate from circulating peripheral blood mononuclear cells which migrate into tissue in the steady state or in response to inflammation. As the most plastic cell of the hemapoetic system, macrophages are classified depending on the milieu and specialization. Macrophages are of various types such as alveolar (lungs), microglia (brain), kupffer cells (hepatic), splenic, intestinal, intraocular (eyes) and bone marrow. Macrophages represent a spectrum of activated phenotypes rather than defined stable subpopulations. During homeostatic conditions, the tissue resident macrophages remain in a quiescent state. Upon requirement, monocytes get recruited and differentiated into macrophages and DCs at the site of inflammation. Mature macrophages can further get polarized into either M1 macrophages (classical activation) or M2 macrophages (alternative activation) and attain their respective phenotypes. They are characterized based on their surface markers, secreted cytokines, nitric oxide enzymes, transcription and epigenetic factors.

Macrophages serve as an effective component of innate immunity for their ability to recognize, engulf and kill potential pathogens. Macrophages are commonly derived from monocytes and play a crucial role in both innate and adaptive immunity [3]. They contribute to the activation of these immune responses by synthesis and secretion of a range of pro-and anti-inflammatory mediators thereby establishing protective immunity. Macrophages also play an important role in the defense system as antimicrobial warriors against invading microbes such as bacteria. Uncontrolled macrophage activity in the host is however noxious and has been linked to various pathogenic conditions such as artherosclerosis, granulomatous disease and macrophage activation syndrome [4-9]. The pivotal role of macrophages during the initiation, regulation and termination of inflammation makes them a major target for the prevention, control and resolution of inflammatory processes in various chronic lung diseases such as chronic obstructive pulmonary disease (COPD) [10-13], asthma [14-16] and idiopathic pulmonary fibrosis (IPF) [17-20].

The alveolar macrophages (AMs) are the predominant leukocyte phenotype in the lung among all age groups (> 89%). Bronchoalveolar lavage (BAL) from healthy adults contains an average of 91% of alveolar macrophages, 7% of lymphocytes, 1% neutrophils and 1% of mast cells [21]. In the lungs, cells of lymphoid origin are sparse when compared to cells derived from the myeloid lineage during an acute immune response. Macrophages initiate phagocytosis and subsequently release cytokines along with other products which orchestrate host cellular defence. Understanding the molecular basis of macrophage polarization is an important aspect to deal with inflammation. The microenvironment plays an important role in the phenotypic polarization of macrophages. This polarization is driven by various factors, signals and diseased conditions. However, the molecular basis of macrophage polarization has not been fully explored. A major question that remains to be answered is about the function of the different macrophage types under various conditions such as steady state, diseased and tissue-repair. The need to understand the polarization of macrophages becomes mandatory in order to improve the therapeutic strategies for different chronic respiratory diseases. In this chapter, the heterogeneity of macrophages, its classification under different conditions, and the status of its polarization in chronic respiratory diseases along with their respective functions are discussed.

2. Monocyte heterogeneity

The mononuclear phagocyte system represents a subgroup of leukocytes described as a population of bone marrow derived CD4+(cluster of differentiation 4) myeloid progenitor cells that circulate in the blood as monocytes [22]. They act as immune effector cells, equipped with chemokine receptors and pathogen recognition receptors on its surface that mediate migration from blood to tissues. These cells do not proliferate in a steady state condition but circulate in blood stream, bone marrow and spleen [23, 24]. They enter the peripheral tissues during inflammation and mature into either macrophages or inflammatory DCs which are significant mediators of inflammatory reaction in the lung tissue. The differentiation of recruited blood monocytes into macrophages depends on the characteristics of inflammation and is also governed by the pulmonary microenvironment. Newly differentiated macrophages can also activate resident macrophages or epithelial cells to secrete more inflammatory cytokines, chemokines and other inflammatory factors which in turn result in more monocyte recruitment to the site of inflammation.

Peripheral-blood monocytes show morphological heterogeneity, such as variability of size, granularity and nuclear morphology [25]. In human blood, monocytes are divided into two subsets depending upon the differential expression of cell surface markers CD14 and CD16, commonly detected by means of cytometry. Monocytes which are $CD14^{hi}$(High) and $CD16^{-}$ (negative) represent the classical subset whereas monocytes with $CD14^{hi}$ and $CD16^{+}$(positive) expression represent the other type characterized by higher expression of major histocompatability complex class II (MHCII) and CD32 antigen [26]. The monocyte heterogeneity in mice is differentiated with the expression of chemokine (C-C motif) receptor 2 (CCR2) and lymphocyte antigen 6 complex (Ly6C). Monocytes which express CCR2, CD62, $CX3CR^{low}$ (chemokine [C-X3-C motif] receptor 1), Ly6C correspond to $CD14^{hi}CD16^{-}$ (classic) human monocytes [27]. Although monocyte heterogeneity is not completely understood, one theory suggests that monocytes continue to develop and mature in the blood and can be recruited into the tissues at various points during maturation continuum [28].

Plasticity is the hallmark of monocytes and it responds to various microenvironmental signals and mount specific phenotypic functional programs. Monocytes in response to the pro-inflammatory signals migrate to the inflamed tissue and differentiate into inflammatory macrophages and DCs. Also in the absence of inflammation, monocytes have been thought to enter the tissues and replenish the pool of tissue resident macrophages and DC populations [29]. However, recent evidences suggest that tissue resident macrophages proliferate and maintain their pool locally, independent of the circulating blood monocytes [30]. However, the precise mechanism for this switch in the role of monocytes from one type to another is not clear. Granulocyte macrophage-colony stimulating factor (GM-CSF) and interleukin 4 (IL4) are able to induce the differentiation of human and mouse monocytes into DCs, irrespective of their subsets [31, 32]. These striking similarities in the characteristic features of mouse and human monocyte subsets establish the conserved mechanisms among the two species. However, since most of our understanding about macrophage biology relies on in vitro studies or severe pathological conditions of animal experimental disease models, one needs to overcome the difficulties in establishing the in vitro and in vivo studies to have a clear mechanistic understanding of the phenotype switching in monocytes under homeostatic conditions. In this context, significant progress has recently been achieved in mice thereby improving our understanding of the weak connection between circulating blood monocytes and resident tissue macrophages. For example it has been shown that AMs originate from fetal monocytes, thus establishing a locally independent, self-maintained pool of highly specialized resident tissue phagocytes. The pool is maintained by local proliferation, mainly triggered by GM-CSF stimulation and under steady state conditions exist independent of replenishment by blood monocytes [30, 33, 34].

3. Populations of macrophages

Macrophages can be derived from circulating monocytes and exhibit a high degree of heterogeneity like their precursors [35, 36]. However, it is still not clear whether in this way differentiated cell will be able to functionally replace resident tissue macrophage. Heterogeneity refers to the ability of macrophages to embark on different phenotypic functional specialization depending upon the anatomical location and its microenvironment. For example, the AMs express high pattern recognition receptors to counter the environmental microbial challenge in the lungs. Likewise, each tissue resident macrophage has its typical functional characterization. It is clear that macrophages represent a spectrum of activated phenotypes rather than discrete stable subpopulation. The main function of immune surveillance remains the same for all the macrophages irrespective of its location. Macrophages play a central role in inflammation and host defence [3] and are characterized by considerable diversity and plasticity [37, 38].

In the lung, distinct macrophage subpopulations have been characterized primarily in infectious disease and asthma models [39-43]. The local conditions present in the lung dictate the differentiation and activation of monocytes and macrophages in addition to the specific developmental pathways [25]. Two unique populations of monocytes are present in circulation. The monocytes enter lungs under steady state conditions and develop into resident tissue interstitial macrophages and AMs [44, 45]. Inflammatory monocytes are recruited in a CCR2-dependent manner at the time of inflammation, and develop into either an activated macrophage population, known as exudative macrophages (ExMacs) or into monocyte-derived dendritic cells (moDCs) [46]. Resident macrophages differ markedly from inflammatory monocyte-derived macrophages in terms of morphology, phenotype, and effector functions [42].

Resident lung interstitial macrophages and AMs express relatively lower MHCII and costimulatory molecules [47]. After activation, they produce low levels of inflammatory cytokines and do not promote T-cell activation. In contrast, ExMacs are a major source of inflammatory cytokines and chemokines, expressing high levels of MHCII and costimulatory molecules. Further, they also stimulate T cell activation [46]. It is hypothesized that ExMacs are recruited to the lung early after noninfectious lung injury and have effector functions distinct from resident macrophages [46]. AMs in the lung provide the first line of defense against inhaled organism and irritants [16, 44]. In addition to their phagocytic role, AMs are known to be a critical modulator of the lung inflammatory response through the production of various pro-inflammatory and anti-inflammatory modulators.

4. Activation and recruitment of macrophages

The presence and evolution of distinct macrophage subsets in the lung serve specific niches in regulating the inflammatory response and its resolution. Based on the patterns of gene expression, protein secretion and roles in host defense mechanisms, macrophages are classified into classically activated macrophages (CAM) and alternatively activated macrophages (AAM). The two main macrophage subsets namely CAM (also termed as M1) and AAM (termed as M2) have been described in analogy to T helper (Th)1 and Th2 lymphocyte archetype activation [3]. In response to various signals, macrophages may undergo M1 classical activation [by toll like receptor (TLR) ligands and interferon gamma (IFNγ)] or M2 alternative activation [by IL4 and IL13]. M1 and M2 activation phenotypes represent two ends of the functional spectrum of macrophage polarization [48] (Figure 1). In addition to these stimulants, various other cytokines and interferons have also been documented in the polarization of macrophages. Addition of transforming growth factor beta 1 (TGFβ1) to monocytes confers the phenotype of leukocytes during in vitro condition [49], whereas exposure to macrophage colony stimulating factors (M-CSF) induces monocytes to differentiate into macrophages under the same condition. Addition of IFNγ [or lipopolysaccharide (LPS)] to M-CSF induces the differentiation of M1-like macrophages whereas addition of IL4 induces the differentiation of M2-like macrophages [50, 51]. A continuum of macrophage polarization is likely to exist beyond these discrete in vitro based classifications [38].

The immune system of alveolar blood barrier in the lungs has to be tightly regulated as pulmonary edema and inflammation can lead to thickening of alveolar walls and thereby compromise gas exchange efficiency [52]. Alveolar macrophages play an important role in maintaining the immune system of the lungs. Multiple subsets of monocyte derived macrophages contribute to distinct stages of inflammation [23, 27]. A fully differentiated macrophage subpopulation can change its phenotype in response to the microenvironment [48, 53, 54]. Each signal from the microenvironment has its specific role in the process of macrophage polarization and the macrophages change their phenotype based on the duration of exposure to the stimulus [53-57]. Macrophages which are exposed to the environment favoring alternative activation, switches its phenotype to M1 when it encounters activation by IFNγ or TNF [58-60]. Various molecules such as 7-oxo-cholesterol (7oxo-C), P50 have been recognized as stimulants of polarization. 7oxo-C has a prominent impact on the phenotype of polarized M1 and M2 macrophages. It stimulates the expression of MHCII by M1 macrophages resulting in upregulation of macrophage function as antigen presenting cells (APC) that favor activation of adaptive immune responses [61]. 7-oxoC affects human macrophage biology by skewing the M1/M2 macrophage balance towards a pro-inflammatory profile. P50 in nuclear factor kappa B (NF-κB) play an essential role in the orientation of macrophage polarization both in vitro and in vivo. This regulatory subunit may play a crucial role in the control of M1 and M2 driven inflammation [62]. Other key transcription factors for polarization are interferon regulatory factor 5 (IRF5), signal transducer and activator of transcription 1 (STAT1) for the M1 and IRF4, STAT6 and peroxisome proliferator activated receptor gamma (PPARγ) for the M2 pathway [63].

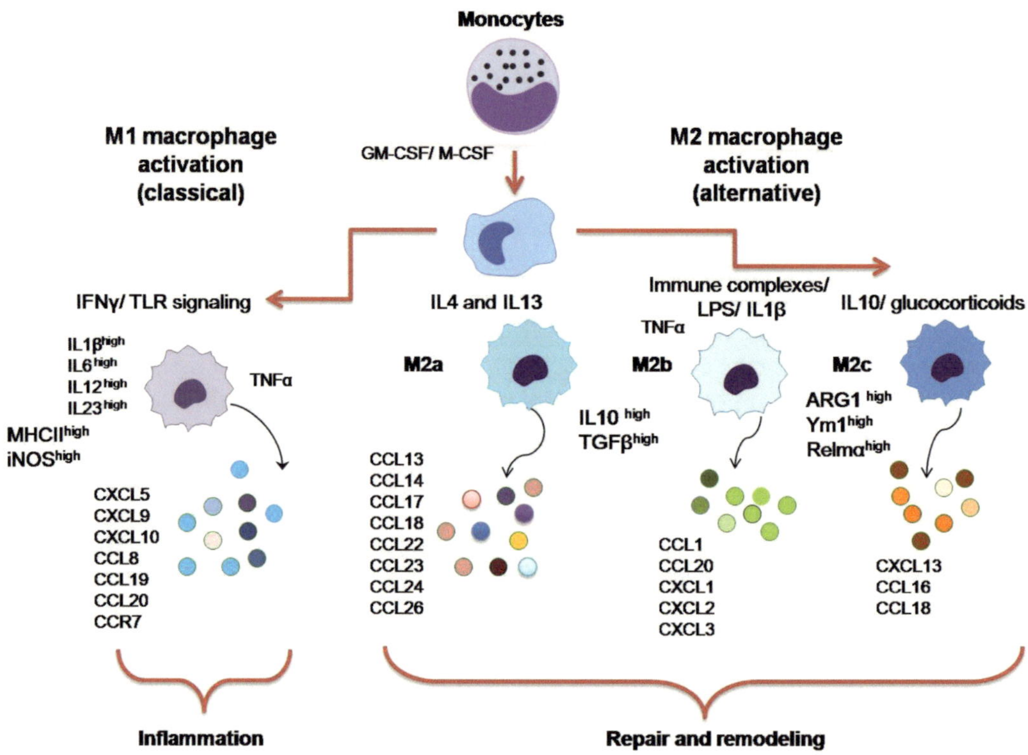

Figure 1. Schematic representation of M1 (classical) and M2 (alternative) macrophage polarization. Several cytokines and chemokines are involved in the classical and alternative activation of macrophages. Monocytes gets differentiated into macrophages which in turn polarize to M1 type on exposure to interferon gamma (IFNγ). Various signals define the different forms of alternative activation of macrophages. Interleukin 4 (IL4) or IL13 induces M2a subtype; IL1β or lipopolysachharide (LPS) or immune compelxes induces M2b macrophages; and IL10 or glucocorticoids results in M2c macrophages [38, 48, 64]. **GM-CSF:** granuloctye macrophage-colony stimulating factor, **M-CSF:** macrophage-colony stimulating factor, **MHCII:** major histocompatibility complex II, **iNOS:** induced nitric oxide synthase, **TNFα:** tumour necrosis factor alpha, **ARG1:** arginase 1, **Ym1:** chitinase-like 3, **Relmα:** resistin like alpha, **CXCL:** chemokine (C-X-C motif) ligand, **CCL:** chemokine (C-C motif) ligand, **CCR:** chemokine (C-C motif) receptor.

5. Classical activation of macrophages (CAM)

M1 macrophages are induced by IFNγ. Other factors which results in the activation of M1 macrophages are LPS, cytokines such as TNFα and GM-CSF. IL12 and IL23 are upregulated while IL10 is down-regulated during M1 macrophage activation [65]. IL1β and TNFα act as inducers as well as effector molecules during this process. It is also observed that Th1 response is involved in classical macrophage activation. M1 macrophage development results in elevated expression of the enzyme induced nitric oxide synthase (iNOS/NOS2) [66] thereby causing production of an excess amount of nitrogen and oxygen intermediates. These cells mediate the resistance against microbes, intracellular parasites and tumours by eliciting tissue disruptive reactions. M1 macrophages, whose prototypical activating stimuli are IFNγ and

LPS, exhibit potent microbicidal properties and promote strong IL12-mediated Th1 responses. M1 macrophages express reduced levels of mannose receptor and Fc receptor for IgG (FcαR)II [67]. Classical polarization of macrophages by cytokines affects lymphocyte proliferation. It also determines the cytokines to be produced by activated macrophages. Pro-inflammatory M1 macrophages release higher amounts of active matrix metalloproteinases (MMPs) such as MMP1 and MMP9 compared to anti-inflammatory M2 cells.

6. Alternate activation of macrophages (AAM)

Macrophages activated in the presence of IL4 are known as alternatively activated macrophages. IL4 along with IL13 are the major cytokines of Th2 immune responses. Macrophages treated with IL4 and IL13 fail to present antigens to T cells and produce low levels of cytokines in vitro [68, 69]. These macrophages are also termed as wound healing and tissue regeneration macrophages because of their ability to produce growth factors contributing to the development of extracellular matrix (ECM). The main properties of M2 like macrophages are expression of higher levels of surface scavenger, mannose and galactose type receptors that are involved in debris clearance. It is worthy to note that although murine M1-and M2-polarized macrophage subsets are relatively easy to distinguish based on combinatorial gene expression profiles, the identification of equivalent subsets in humans is a more challenging task [61]. There are various forms of AAM [70]. Immune complexes along with IL10, glucocorticoids activate M2 macrophages besides IL4 and IL13. Contrary to the M1 macrophages, during polarization IL12 and IL23 are released at lower levels whereas scavenger, mannose and galactose-type receptors are expressed at higher levels. IL4 was initially believed to act as anti-inflammatory for its ability to suppress TNFα and IL6 production in macrophages. AAMs also downregulate host protection against selected pathogens, but promote parasite encapsulation.

There are three distinct subtypes of AAMs namely M2a, M2b and M2c (Figure 1). This classification is mainly based upon the interaction between the specific ligands and receptors of the macrophages. The subtypes of AAMs are characterized based on the cell surface markers and specialization. Low amounts of IL4 promote a Th2 cell response. If the stimulus persists, it results in sufficient production of IL13, which is a dominant Th2 effector cell cytokine. IL13 in turn induces responses in both hemapoietic and non-hemapoietic cells. The diversity of macrophage function is indicated by their polarized states, distinct subpopulations and localization in the lung. Signals inducing M2 polarization downregulate the activities of NF-κB and STAT1. IL4 and IL13 selectively induce CCL24, CCL17, CCL18 and CCL22 in M2a macrophages with inhibition by IFNγ [70]. M2b macrophages express high levels of IL10 and low levels of IL12. M2c macrophages express high levels of CXCL13, CCL16 and CCL18 [70]. Unlike other discrete leukocyte populations, macrophages maintain their plasticity and can alter their phenotype based on the microenvironment, including the cytokine milieu among the other factors. Importantly, M1 cells can repolarize towards M2 after the phagocytosis of apoptotic neutrophils [71, 72] suggesting that reprogramming of inflammatory macrophage towards M2 phenotype may be involved in the resolution phase of acute lung injury.

The markers of polarized macrophage were originally identified by Becker and colleagues using membrane proteomics of macrophages [73]. AM induces high IL10 production and also weakly express the surface receptors for M2 cells. This suggests that an early recruitment or activation of a resident population can serve to balance the pro-inflammatory milieu. A population of pro-inflammatory M1 cells within the interstitium is also found to be resident cells. During the resolution phase of lung injury, this population (CD11b^{low} and CD45^{hi}) up regulates the M2 markers, transferrin receptor (TFRC), chitinase –like 3 (YM1) and arginase 1 (ARG1) expression representing M1 cells in transition. A similar trend of repolarization markers is observed among these cells located in the alveolar space. CD11b^{hi} expressing population of cells demonstrates higher iNOS, IL12 and ARG1 gene expression. This subpopulation coexpressing iNos and ARG1 may be regarded as representative cells which share M1 and M2 markers [74]. The CD11b^{hi} cells also express high amounts of IL12, another factor by which these cells can regulate T cell responses. Cu, Zn superoxide dismutase (Cu, Zn-SOD) polarize the macrophages to M2 phenotype, and Cu, Zn-SOD-mediated H_2O_2 levels modulates M2 gene expression at the transcriptional level by redox regulation of a critical cysteine in STAT6 [75].

7. Resident alveolar macrophages (AM)

The lung provides an appropriate example of macrophage heterogeneity within an organ and effects of the microenvironment on the respective functions of macrophages located within that particular environment. Based on the anatomical location within the lung, there are three types of macrophages viz., alveolar, interstitial, and the intravascular macrophages. Each macrophage performs specific functions, as for example, the primary function of alveolar macrophage is the removal of particulates and microorganisms from the alveolar space. The pulmonary intravascular macrophages perform the same function but in the circulation whereas the interstitial macrophages might have a role in limiting inflammation, fibrosis, and antigen presentation [76, 77]. However, the role of macrophage heterogeneity in development of various macrophage population and its subsets is not clearly understood. As described above, resident alveolar macrophages are derived from fetal monocytes but not blood monocytes. However, it is still not clear whether the ExMacs are differentiated after inflammation from recruited monocytes can actually replace those developed under steady state conditions. Further, it remains unclear whether resident macrophages in the respective tissue niche are terminally differentiated or remain flexible to change their phenotype from one niche to another according to the respective signals and microenvironment.

In summary AMs are an unique type of mononuclear phagocytes that populate the surface of the lung in steady state. It forms the first line of defence against foreign particles invading the alveolar space. AMs get activated on pathogen recognition, thereby releasing early response cytokines such as TNFα and IL1 β. The early response also stimulate the neighboring alveolar cells to produce chemokines. These chemokines mediate the recruitment of neutrophils, ExMacs and lymphoctyes [78, 79]. AMs contribute to respiratory tolerance by inducing Fox3 expression in naïve T cells [80]. Noteworthy, the bone marrow with derived blood monocytes does not significantly contribute to the alveolar macrophage compartment during steady state conditions. Previous alveolar macrophage half-life studies were confounded by the facts that they did not account for the inflammatory and stimulatory effects of irradiation conditioning regimens [79].

8. Molecular basis of macrophage polarization

Macrophage polarization is associated with significant changes at the transcriptional level, although the two polarizing conditions are very different. M1 polarization profoundly affects the transcriptional profile while M2 polarization results in only subtle adjustments [65]. The investigations on the transcriptional events associated with M-CSF-dependent monocyte-to-macrophage differentiation and subsequent M1 or M2 polarization induced by LPS and IFNγ or IL4 demonstrated the existence of a complex network of gene regulation. Modulation of genes involved in general cellular metabolic activities is a prominent feature of macrophage differentiation and polarization. The enzymes such as sphingosine 1 phosphate and ceramide 1 phosphate are used to distinguish the polarized forms of macrophages as sphingosine and ceramide kinase are selectively present in M1 and M2 macrophages respectively [65].

Classically activated macrophages include prototypic M1 polarization markers, such as the indoleamine-pyrrole 2,3 dioxygenase, the lysosomal associated membrane protein 3, IL7R and CCR7 [81]. Classically activated macrophages are characterized by increased expression of the solute carrier family member SLC21A15 and SLC31A2, while alternatively activated macrophages exhibit increased SLC4A7, SLC38A6 expression. In case of humans, membrane expression of the markers CD80 and CD200R are specific for M1 and M2 polarized macrophages respectively whereas mannose receptor (CD206) expression does not vary between M1 and M2. Transcript analysis further identified six markers of M1 polarization [IL-12p35, CXCL10, CXCL11, CCL5, CCR7 and indoleamine 2,3-dioxygenase 1 (IDO1)]; five markers of M2 polarization [TGFβ, CCL14, CCL22, scavenger receptor class B, member 1 (SCARB1)] and several transcription factors IRF4, IRF5, STAT1, STAT6 and PPARγ] involved in macrophage polarization. Ability of human M-CSF generated macrophage to polarize toward M1 or M2 subtype is also associated with enhanced secretion of TNFα, IL1β, IL12p40, CXCL10 and IL10 (for M1); or CCL22 (for M2). Moreover, the comparison of the expression of M1 markers in M-CSF and GM-CSF macrophages polarized towards M1 subtype has revealed similarities [82].

Chemokine receptors are differentially expressed on polarized Th cells. Typically, CXCR3 and CCR5 are preferentially expressed on polarized Th1 cells, whereas CCR3, CCR4 and CCR8 have been associated with the Th2 phenotypes. Distinct chemokines are associated with M1 and the various forms of M2 macrophage activation. LPS and IFNγ induce the expression of CXCL10, CXCL9 and CCL5 [83-85]. In addition, LPS mediates induction of the CXCL10, CXCL9 and CCL5 genes through the activation of the transcription factor IRF3, which results in IFNγ expression and subsequent STAT1 activation [85]. Further, LPS activation of monocytes or macrophages results in the NF-κB dependent transcription of inflammatory chemokines such as CXCL1,2,3,5,8,9 and 10; and CCL2, 3,4,5,11,17 and 22 [86]. Resistin like alpha (Relmα),

YM1 are also expressed in higher levels and are used as phenotypic markers for M2 polarized macrophages. CCL13, CCL14, CCL17, CCL18 and CCL24 [87] are specifically induced in M2a macrophages [64, 88], whereas M2b macrophages rather characterized by expression of high levels of CCL20, CXCL1, CXCL2 and CXCL3; whereas M2c macrophages express high levels of CXCL13, CCL16 and CCL18 [64].

9. T cells and Alveolar macrophages

T cell mediated immunity is important in the lung in order to protect the host from inhaled pathogens and environmental antigens [89-91]. Furthermore, most of the environmental antigens encountered by the lung are innocuous. Hence it is crucial for the resident immune cells to distinguish such inert antigens from those derived from pathogens and respond appropriately. The immunoregulatory mechanisms employed by the lung include the components for surfactant lining [92], products secreted by alveolar type II epithelial cells as well as alveolar macrophages which altogether actively suppress T cell proliferation. Moreover, AM induces anergy (immune unresponsiveness) in T cells which is reversible upon its removal from culture [91]. T cells isolated from lungs of rodents express low levels of IL2 receptor (IL2R/CD25) [91]. The Immunoregulators associated with AM include prostaglandins, leukotrienes, IL1 and nitric oxide [89]. AMs also downregulate local pulmonary immune responses against intratracheally administered T cell dependent antigens [93].

AMs from rat, mouse and human differ markedly in its potency to inhibit mitogen-induced T cell proliferation. However, T cells stimulated in the presence of AMs display a similar phenotype in all species examined, i.e. CD3 downregulation, upregulation of IL2R, increased IL2 production and inability to respond to IL2 [94]. Thus, AMs appear to allow T cell activation and effector functions, while selectively inhibiting T cell proliferation. The suppressive activity of AMs is restricted to the final step in the activation process, (i.e. proliferation). Through CD3 downregulation, IL2R expression and IL2 secretion appear to proceed normally [94].

T cells from humans produce less IL2 than autologous blood-derived T cells [95]. FoxP3 is a master regulator of regulatory T cells (Treg). FoxP3 expression is regarded as definitive marker for cells with regulatory function in mice and humans [96, 97]. AMs obtained from BAL of mice or humans enhance FoxP3 expression in CD4+FoxP3-T cells in vitro. Activation of naïve T cells in the presence of either AMs or AM-conditioned media prevents T cell proliferation. This effect can be reversed by inhibiting binding of retinoic acid to its receptor or by blocking TGFβ1 signaling [80]. AMs induce intracellular FoxP3 expression in CD4+T cells. It promotes IL10 while suppressing IFNγ production by the same T cell in vitro [80]. AMs induce an immune unresponsiveness in T cells and also affects its proliferation.

10. Role of macrophages in chronic respiratory diseases

Macrophages have the ability to elicit an immune response and resolve the inflammatory processes. The macrophages of the respiratory system are involved in the pathogenesis of different respiratory diseases such as COPD, asthma and pulmonary fibrosis. Different phenotypes of macrophages are involved in these respiratory diseases which play an important role in either inflammation and / or resolution process.

11. Chronic obstructive pulmonary disease (COPD)

COPD is a global epidemic, mainly caused by cigarette smoke exposure (smokers disease) and high particulate air pollution (as associated to in-house cooking) with an alarming increase in its mortality rate [98]. COPD is characterized by an inflammatory airway obstruction and loss of alveolar tissue thereby causing reduced respiratory surface area (emphysema). Macrophages are elevated and accumulate in small airways, bronchioles and alveoli during COPD irrespective of the disease severity. Macrophages monitor and respond to their microenvironment that can define tissue remodelling and possibly control other inflammatory events. AMs in the lung are an important source of both proteinases and antiproteinases. They secrete a series MMPs (1,9 and 12) [10, 99-101] and tissue inhibitor of metalloproteinases (TIMPs). In addition, they also secrete lysosomal cysteine proteinases [Cathepsin K, L, S (CTSK, CTSL and CTSS respectively)] and their inhibitor cystatin C (CST3) [10, 102]. An imbalance between proteinase and antiproteinase is considered to be an important event in the pathogenesis of COPD [103].

Macrophage derived MMPs as well as cathepsins are elastinolytic [10, 102, 104] and are important in airway inflammation and development of emphysema [9, 10, 101].Elastinolysis, an essential event of emphysema [105] results in the destruction of lung tissues during COPD [106, 107]. AMs have also been shown to release neutrophil elastase in vitro [102, 108]. There is a positive association between macrophage numbers in the alveolar walls and the presence of mild to moderate emphysema as well as the degree of small airways disease in patients with COPD [109, 110]. Dysregulated expression of macrophage MMPs either directly or indirectly by cigarette smoke exposure can lead to lung parenchyma destruction, characteristic of emphysema.

The role of different subsets of AMs in the pathogensis of COPD is yet to be fully ascertained. Increased expression of iNos in AMs is found in patients with COPD [111-113]. Smoke exposure enhances the release of pro-inflammatory cytokines such as IL1β, IL6, IL8 and TNFα [114-118] in the lungs which are markers of M1 macrophage polarization. There is also contradictory transcriptome based evidence that M2 polarized alveolar macrophage may contribute to COPD pathogenesis [119]. Further, COPD exacerbation, characterized by severe shortness of breath, is a common occurrence, which is usually caused due to an infection or exposure to environmental pollutants. Impaired phagocytosis, a characteristic feature of M1 polarized macrophages is also considered to be an important cause for increased COPD severity [120]. Analysis of BAL fluid of COPD patients suggests that smoking cessation partly changes the macrophage polarization from a pro-inflammatory M1 towards an anti-inflammatory M2 macrophage phenotype [121]. M2 polarized alveolar macrophage have been shown to produce MMP12 which plays an important role in cigarette smoke induced emphysema

[122-124]. It could be considered that COPD pathogenesis is largely contributed by dysfunction of macrophages rather than a single subset of AMs.

12. Asthma

Asthma is characterized by airway inflammation and airway hyperresponsiveness (AHR). Macrophages also contribute significantly to the development of asthma [125]. The inflammatory process of asthma is dominated by Th2 inflammation, but there is also involvement of both types M1 and M2 macrophages [14]. The balance between different phenotypes of macrophages changes with the severity of asthma [126]. In case of acute exacerbation of chronic asthma, AMs are found to significantly enhance the expression of AAM markers along with pro-inflammatory cytokines (IFNγ and TNFα) and cell surface proteins. Ironically, the cell surface proteins associated with antigen presentation are M1 inducers [127, 128]. Elevated serum IFNγ correlates with the severity of airway inflammation in atopic asthma, and IFNγ has been linked to mechanisms inducing AHR [129]. It was demonstrated that IL33/ST2 plays a significant role in the amplification of AAM polarization and chemokine production which contribute to innate and Ag-induced airway inflammation [130].

The ability of AMs to phagocytose apoptotic cells is known as efferocytosis. Macrophage efferocytosis is impaired in non-eosinophilic asthma to a similar degree as in COPD [131]. In mice with less severe asthma, M1 macrophage numbers were higher and correlated negatively with M2 macrophage counts. Lower numbers of M2-like macrophages were found in mice exposed to house dust mites. The balance between macrophage phenotypes changes as the severity of allergic airway inflammation increases. Influencing this imbalanced relationship could be a novel approach to treat asthma [126]. CCL18 and YKL40 (chitinase 3-like 1) levels and CHIT1 (chitinase 1) activity are enhanced in allergic airway inflammation and thus may contribute to airway remodelling in asthma [132]. M2 macrophages play a role in eosinophil and potentially other leukocyte migration patterns into asthmatic airways [133]. Dysregulation of alveolar macrophage function results in dendritic cell-mediated mechanisms of allergic airway inflammation [134]. AMs can also contribute to the genetic susceptibility to allergic asthma [39].

13. Pulmonary fibrosis

Fibrosis is the result of persistent or dysregulated wound healing, usually in response to some type of repeated injury. It is often associated with chronic inflammation, alveolar epithelial hyperplasia and excessive deposition of ECM [135]. Lung macrophages and circulating monocytes play an important role during pulmonary fibrosis. AMs are involved in the removal of accumulated collagen. AAM play an important role in the development and resolution of lung fibrosis after injury, but their growth promoting activity raise the intriguing possibility that persistent M2 activity might contribute to the failure in resolving fibrosis in IPF patients.

Sun and coworkers [136] reported that increased numbers of AAMs induced by over expression of IL10 results in induction of lung fibrosis in mice. Accordingly increased expression of CD206 (another marker of AAM) and IL4 is observed in patients with IPF and systemic sclerosis [137, 138]. Secretion of IL4 and IL13 by T cells is required for fibroblast migration and proliferation and their subsequent differentiation into myofibroblasts. IFNγ, in contrast, attenuates the fibrotic response and induces collagen degradation [139]. Paired immunoglobulin like receptor beta (PIRB) contributes to the pathogenesis of pulmonary fibrosis via the negative regulation of macrophage effector function and fibrogenic mediator expression. PIRB negatively regulates IL4-induced macrophage activation. Various studies have also demonstrated the role of AAM production in pulmonary fibrosis [140]. Relmα, a hallmark M2 macrophage marker is upregulated in pulmonary fibrosis which is controlled by IL4/ IL13-and STAT6-dependent pathways [141].

The Th2 cytokines IL4 and IL13, like TGFβ1, directly stimulate collagen synthesis in mouse and human fibroblasts [142]. They also promote the development of the classic myofibroblast phenotype in human lung fibroblasts [143]. Macrophages accumulate in areas of fibrotic injury but their role remains incompletely understood. A study using silica-induced model of lung fibrosis found that the IL4Rα-dependent differentiation of AAM is critical for the induction and maintenance of the CD4^{+}Th2 response required to trigger fibrosis [144]. Chitotriosidase, an enzyme especially expressed by M2 macrophages is also overexpressed in patients with IPF, especially in a progressing stage suggesting that this enzyme plays a role in the pathogenesis of diffuse lung disease-associated fibrosis [145, 146].

Polarization of macrophages to the M1 phenotype attenuates pulmonary fibrosis [65]. Fibrosis may be independent of monocyte and lung macrophage activity during the inflammation phase of bleomycin injury, a frequently used animal model for IPF. The depletion of lung macrophages during the inflammatory phase of bleomycin injury has no effect on the early as well as peak stage of lung fibrosis. However, during the progressive phase, lung macrophage depletion reduces the degree of pulmonary fibrosis. Depletion of lung macrophages during the resolution phase of bleomycin induced lung fibrosis slowed down the process [147]. Macrophages may promote resolution during the reversible phase of bleomycin induced pulmonary fibrosis [148]. Overexpression of MMP9 by AMs has the capability to attenuate the fibrosis induced by bleomycin [149]. ExMacs are recruited to the lung after noninfectious injury by bleomycin and are the major source of macrophages derived CXCL10 [46]. ExMacs are CD11c^{+}, MHCII^{in} Gr-1 int and are separated from resident AMs by high expression of both CD11b and CX3CR1. Everson and colleagues [147] separated AMs into 18 density defined subpopulations. Bleomycin altered the proportions of these subpopulations and enhanced the production of TNFα production in these specific subpopulations. Bleomycin-treated *Pirb*$^{(-/-)}$ mice displayed an increased expression of collagen and IL4 associated profibrogenic markers Relmα, MMP12, TIMP1, and osteopontin, which were localized to AMs. Thus, macrophages may have a role in resolution during the reversible phase of bleomycin induced pulmonary fibrosis [148].

14. Environmental exposure to particle inhalation

Epidemiologic and occupational studies show that exposure to high concentrations of ambient particulate matter cause cardiopulmonary health effects, including exacerbation of pre-existing lung disease as well as the development of respiratory infections. Particle related oxidative stress and inflammatory responses are considered to be key for the subsequent health effects, but the precise mechanism how inhaled poorly soluble, sterile, endotoxin free particle induce pulmonary inflammation is not well understood [150]. Since the size of the inhaled material determines their penetration depth into the lungs, smaller particle (<100nm) cause higher alveolar lung burden than bigger sized particles. Lung surface macrophages (i.e. AMs) do not efficiently phagocytose small, sub-100nm sized, so called ultrafine particles (UFP) or nanoparticles (NP), but take them up in a rather sporadic and unspecific way [151]. But the evidence that UFP bypass the most important clearance mechanism for particles deposited in the alveoli, namely phagocytic uptake by macrophages, requires further clarification as to whether these results are specific for the material, the size or other characteristics of the particles. A rethinking of clearance pathways for inhaled UFP is therefore considered necessary [151].

Inhalation of ultrafine carbon particles triggers a biphasic pro-inflammatory process in the lung, involving the activation of macrophages and the upregulation of immunomodulatory proteins [152]. Higher doses cause a distinct inflammatory response characterized by the release of pro-inflammatory cytokines and accumulation of inflammatory leukocytes [153]. A single exposure to these carbon particles however causes only a transient inflammatory response, which resolves within one week after treatment [154]. Black carbon laden AMs however are observed even at much later time points when no inflammatory stimulation in the lungs is detectable. Whether the immunological activity of these long-living tissue macrophages gets changed remains unknown. In animal experiments, when lung inflammation for example is induced by titanium di oxide (TiO2) particles in rats, AMs induce the production of IL-13 and IL-25 production. This in turn modulates the inflammatory response [155]. When exposed to gold NPs, it is found that AMs efficiently internalize NPs by endocytosis, and rearrangements of vesicles and of NPs within the vesicles of macrophages occurred [156]. The uptake of gold particles by AMs is limited, though to a low degree, systemic particle translocation is reported. To summarise, inhaled NPs or UFPs pose high burden to the integrity of lungs as these particles penetrate into the susceptible alveolar region due to the ineffective clearance mechanisms. Whether an activation of lung macrophages, potentially caused by particle-cell interactions, results in a change of their immunological properties thereby increasing the susceptibility for secondary infection warrants further investigations.

15. Conclusion

Macrophages are essential to host defense mechanism. The alveolar macrophages exhibit unique properties, including uncharacteristic phenotypic features, remarkable plasticity and functionality. Various factors of the lung microenvironment define the polarization of macrophages. The temporal changes in the polarization of macrophages during chronic pulmonary diseases help in the regulation of tissue repair and remodeling. Thus understanding of the molecular mechanisms and microenvironment biology of macrophage polarization is a crucial step in evolving novel therapeutic strategies for treating chronic respiratory diseases.

Acknowledgements

(S.U.) CSIR-SRA (13-8553A)-2012/POOL

Author details

Leema George[1], Swapna Upadhyay[2], Koustav Ganguly[1] and Tobias Stoeger[3*]

*Address all correspondence to: tobias.stoeger@helmholtz-muenchen.de

1 SRM Research Institute, SRM University, Chennai, India

2 Department of Biotechnology, Indian Institute of Technology, Madras, Chennai, India

3 Institute of Lung Biology and Disease, Comprehensive Pneumology Center, Helmholtz Zentrum Munich, German Research Center for Environmental Health, Munich, Germany

KG; TS: Equal contribution

References

[1] Occupational and Enviromental Health. Fifth edition ed. Levy BS, Wegman DH, Baron SL, Sokas RK, editors: Lippincott Williams and Wilkins; 2006.

[2] Hubeau C, Puchelle E, Gaillard D. Distinct Pattern of Immune Cell Population in the Lung of Human Fetuses with Cystic Fibrosis. Journal of Allergy and Clinical Immunology. 2001;108(4):524-529.

[3] Gordon S, Martinez F. Alternative Activation of Macrophages: Mechanism and Functions. Immunity. 2010;32(5):593-604.

[4] Grom AA, Mellins ED. Macrophage Activation Syndrome: Advances Towards Understanding Pathogenesis. Current Opinion in Rheumatology. 2010;22(5):561-566.

[5] Heymann F, Trautwein C, Tacke F. Monocytes and Macrophages as Cellular Targets in Liver Fibrosis. Inflammation and Allergy Drug Targets. 2009;8(4):307-318.

[6] Sohn JJ, Schetter AJ, Yfantis HG, Ridnour LA, Horikawa I, Khan MA, Robles AI, Hussain SP, Goto A, Bowman ED, Hofseth LJ, Bartkova J, Bartek J, Wogan GN, Wink DA, Harris CC. Macrophages, Nitric Oxide and Micrornas Are Associated with DNA Damage Response Pathway and Senescence in Inflammatory Bowel Disease. PLoS One. 2012;7(9):e44156.

[7] Murray PJ, Wynn TA. Protective and Pathogenic Functions of Macrophage Subsets. Nature Reviews Immunology. 2011;11(11):723-737.

[8] Libby P, Ridker PM, Hansson GK. Progress and Challenges in Translating the Biology of Atherosclerosis. Nature. 2011;473(7347):317-325.

[9] Shalhoub J, Falck-Hansen MA, Davies AH, Monaco C. Innate Immunity and Monocyte-Macrophage Activation in Atherosclerosis. Journal of inflammation (London, England). 2011;8:9.

[10] Shapiro S. The Macrophage in Chronic Obstructive Pulmonary Disease. American Journal of Respiratory and Critical Care Medicine. 1999;160:S29-S32.

[11] Tetley TD. Macrophages and the Pathogenesis of Copd. Chest. 2002;121(5 Suppl): 156S-159S.

[12] Barnes PJ. Mediators of Chronic Obstructive Pulmonary Disease. Pharmacological Reviews. 2004;56(4):515-548.

[13] Brusselle G, Joos G, Bracke K. New Insights into the Immunology of Chronic Obstructive Pulmonary Disease. Lancet. 2011;378(9795):1015-1026.

[14] Balhara J, Gounni AS. The Alveolar Macrophages in Asthma: A Double-Edged Sword. Mucosal Immunology. 2012;5(6):605-609.

[15] Yang M, Kumar R, Hansbro P, Foster P. Emerging Roles of Pulmonary Macrophages in Driving the Development of Severe Asthma. Journal of Leukocyte Biology. 2012;91(4):557-569.

[16] Marc P-G. The Alveolar Macrophage. American Journal of Respiratory Cell and Molecular Biology. 2004;31.

[17] Nuovo GJ, Hagood JS, Magro CM, Chin N, Kapil R, Davis L, Marsh CB, Folcik VA. The Distribution of Immunomodulatory Cells in the Lungs of Patients with Idiopathic Pulmonary Fibrosis. Modern Pathology. 2012;25(3):416-433.

[18] Rydell-Törmänen K, Andréasson K, Hesselstrand R, Risteli J, Heinegård D, Saxne T, Westergren-Thorsson G. Extracellular Matrix Alterations and Acute Inflammation; Developing in Parallel During Early Induction of Pulmonary Fibrosis. Laboratory Investigation. 2012;92(6):917-925.

[19] Wynn T, Barron L. Macrophages: Master Regulators of Inflammation and Fibrosis. Seminars in liver disease. 2010;30(3):245-257.

[20] Homer R, Elias J, Lee C, Herzog E. Modern Concepts on the Role of Inflammation in Pulmonary Fibrosis. Archives of Pathology and Laboratory Medicine. 2011;135(6): 780-788.

[21] Olsen HH, Grunewald J, Tornling G, Sköld CM, Eklund A. Bronchoalveolar Lavage Results Are Independent of Season, Age, Gender and Collection Site. PLoS One. 2012;7(8):e43644.

[22] van Furth R, Cohn ZA. The Origin and Kinetics of Mononuclear Phagocytes. Journal of Experimental Medicine. 1968;128(3):415-435.

[23] Auffray C, Sieweke MH, Geissmann F. Blood Monocytes: Development, Heterogeneity, and Relationship with Dendritic Cells. Annual Review of Immunology. 2009;27:669-692.

[24] Swirski FK, Nahrendorf M, Etzrodt M, Wildgruber M, Cortez-Retamozo V, Panizzi P, Figueiredo JL, Kohler RH, Chudnovskiy A, Waterman P, Aikawa E, Mempel TR, Libby P, Weissleder R, Pittet MJ. Identification of Splenic Reservoir Monocytes and Their Deployment to Inflammatory Sites. Science. 2009;325(5940):612-616.

[25] Gordon S, Taylor PR. Monocyte and Macrophage Heterogeneity. Nature Reviews. Immunology. 2005;5(12):953-964.

[26] Passlick B, Flieger D, Ziegler-Heitbrock HW. Identification and Characterization of a Novel Monocyte Subpopulation in Human Peripheral Blood. Blood. 1989;74(7): 2527-2534.

[27] Geissmann F, Jung S, Littman DR. Blood Monocytes Consist of Two Principal Subsets with Distinct Migratory Properties. Immunity. 2003;19(1):71-82.

[28] Sunderkotter C, Nikolic T, Dillon MJ, Van Rooijen N, Stehling M, Drevets DA, Leenen PJ. Subpopulations of Mouse Blood Monocytes Differ in Maturation Stage and Inflammatory Response. The Journal of Immunology. 2004;172(7):4410-4417.

[29] Gordon S, Taylor P. Monocyte and Macrophage Heterogeneity. Nature reviews. Immunology. 2005;5(12):953-964.

[30] Hashimoto D, Chow A, Noizat C, Teo P, Beasley MB, Leboeuf M, Becker CD, See P, Price J, Lucas D, Greter M, Mortha A, Boyer SW, Forsberg EC, Tanaka M, van Rooijen N, Garcia-Sastre A, Stanley ER, Ginhoux F, Frenette PS, Merad M. Tissue-Resident Macrophages Self-Maintain Locally Throughout Adult Life with Minimal Contribution from Circulating Monocytes. Immunity. 2013;38(4):792-804.

[31] Sallusto F, Lanzavecchia A. Efficient Presentation of Soluble Antigen by Cultured Human Dendritic Cells Is Maintained by Granulocyte/Macrophage Colony-Stimulat-

ing Factor Plus Interleukin 4 and Downregulated by Tumor Necrosis Factor Alpha. Journal of Experimental Medicine. 1994;179(4):1109-1118.

[32] Geissmann F, Auffray C, Palframan R, Wirrig C, Ciocca A, Campisi L, Narni-Mancinelli E, Lauvau G. Blood Monocytes: Distinct Subsets, How They Relate to Dendritic Cells, and Their Possible Roles in the Regulation of T-Cell Responses. Immunology and Cell Biology. 2008;86(5):398-408.

[33] Yona S, Kim KW, Wolf Y, Mildner A, Varol D, Breker M, Strauss-Ayali D, Viukov S, Guilliams M, Misharin A, Hume DA, Perlman H, Malissen B, Zelzer E, Jung S. Fate Mapping Reveals Origins and Dynamics of Monocytes and Tissue Macrophages under Homeostasis. Immunity. 2013;38(1):79-91.

[34] Guilliams M, De Kleer I, Henri S, Post S, Vanhoutte L, De Prijck S, Deswarte K, Malissen B, Hammad H, Lambrecht BN. Alveolar Macrophages Develop from Fetal Monocytes That Differentiate into Long-Lived Cells in the First Week of Life Via Gm-Csf. Journal of Experimental Medicine. 2013;210(10):1977-1992.

[35] Dijkstra CD, Van Vliet E, Dopp EA, van der Lelij AA, Kraal G. Marginal Zone Macrophages Identified by a Monoclonal Antibody: Characterization of Immuno-and Enzyme-Histochemical Properties and Functional Capacities. Immunology. 1985;55(1): 23-30.

[36] Kraal G, Janse M. Marginal Metallophilic Cells of the Mouse Spleen Identified by a Monoclonal Antibody. Immunology. 1986;58(4):665-669.

[37] Sica A, Larghi P, Mancino A, Rubino L, Porta C, Totaro MG, Rimoldi M, Biswas SK, Allavena P, Mantovani A. Macrophage Polarization in Tumour Progression. Semin Cancer Biol. 2008;18(5):349-355.

[38] Sica A, Mantovani A. Macrophage Plasticity and Polarization: In Vivo Veritas. The Journal of Clinical Investigation. 2012;122(3):787-795.

[39] Careau E, Bissonnette EY. Adoptive Transfer of Alveolar Macrophages Abrogates Bronchial Hyperresponsiveness. American Journal of Respiratory Cell and Molecular Biology. 2004;31(1):22-27.

[40] Lensmar C, Elmberger G, Sandgren P, Skold CM, Eklund A. Leukocyte Counts and Macrophage Phenotypes in Induced Sputum and Bronchoalveolar Lavage Fluid from Normal Subjects. The European Respiratory Journal. 1998;12(3):595-600.

[41] Liang J, Jung Y, Tighe R, Xie T, Liu N, Leonard M, Gunn M, Jiang D, Noble P. A Macrophage Subpopulation Recruited by Cc Chemokine Ligand-2 Clears Apoptotic Cells in Noninfectious Lung Injury. American Journal of Physiology. Lung Cellular and Molecular Physiology. 2012;302(9):40.

[42] Maus U, Janzen S, Wall G, Srivastava M, Blackwell T, Christman J, Seeger W, Welte T, Lohmeyer J. Resident Alveolar Macrophages Are Replaced by Recruited Mono-

cytes in Response to Endotoxin-Induced Lung Inflammation. American Journal of Respiratory Cell and Molecular Biology. 2006;35(2):227-235.

[43] Spiteri MA, Clarke SW, Poulter LW. Isolation of Phenotypically and Functionally Distinct Macrophage Subpopulations from Human Bronchoalveolar Lavage. The European Respiratory Journal. 1992;5(6):717-726.

[44] Guth AM, Janssen WJ, Bosio CM, Crouch EC, Henson PM, Dow SW. Lung Environment Determines Unique Phenotype of Alveolar Macrophages. American Journal of Physiology Lung Cellular and Molecular Physiology. 2009;296.

[45] Lohmann-Matthes ML, Steinmuller C, Franke-Ullmann G. Pulmonary Macrophages. The European Respiratory Journal. 1994;7(9):1678-1689.

[46] Tighe RM, Liang J, Liu N, Jung Y, Jiang D, Gunn MD, Noble PW. Recruited Exudative Macrophages Selectively Produce Cxcl10 after Noninfectious Lung Injury. American Journal of Respiratory Cell and Molecular Biology. 2011;45(4):781-788.

[47] Lee HW, Choi HJ, Ha SJ, Lee KT, Kwon YG. Recruitment of Monocytes/Macrophages in Different Tumor Microenvironments. Biochimica et Biophysica Acta. 2013;1835(2): 170-179.

[48] Mosser D, Edwards J. Exploring the Full Spectrum of Macrophage Activation. Nature reviews. Immunology. 2008;8(12):958-969.

[49] Geissmann F, Prost C, Monnet JP, Dy M, Brousse N, Hermine O. Transforming Growth Factor Beta1, in the Presence of Granulocyte/Macrophage Colony-Stimulating Factor and Interleukin 4, Induces Differentiation of Human Peripheral Blood Monocytes into Dendritic Langerhans Cells. Journal of Experimental Medicine. 1998;187(6):961-966.

[50] Stein M, Keshav S, Harris N, Gordon S. Interleukin 4 Potently Enhances Murine Macrophage Mannose Receptor Activity: A Marker of Alternative Immunologic Macrophage Activation. Journal of Experimental Medicine. 1992;176(1):287-292.

[51] Martinez FO, Helming L, Gordon S. Alternative Activation of Macrophages: An Immunologic Functional Perspective. Annual Review of Immunology. 2009;27:451-483.

[52] Lambrecht BN. Alveolar Macrophage in the Driver's Seat. Immunity. 2006;24(4): 366-368.

[53] Stout RD, Jiang C, Matta B, Tietzel I, Watkins SK, Suttles J. Macrophages Sequentially Change Their Functional Phenotype in Response to Changes in Microenvironmental Influences. The Journal of Immunology. 2005;175(1):342-349.

[54] Stout RD, Suttles J. Immunosenescence and Macrophage Functional Plasticity: Dysregulation of Macrophage Function by Age-Associated Microenvironmental Changes. Immunological Reviews. 2005;205:60-71.

[55] Goerdt S, Orfanos CE. Other Functions, Other Genes: Alternative Activation of Antigen-Presenting Cells. Immunity. 1999;10(2):137-142.

[56] Gratchev A, Kzhyshkowska J, Kothe K, Muller-Molinet I, Kannookadan S, Utikal J, Goerdt S. Mphi1 and Mphi2 Can Be Re-Polarized by Th2 or Th1 Cytokines, Respectively, and Respond to Exogenous Danger Signals. Immunobiology. 2006;211(6-8): 473-486.

[57] Biswas SK, Sica A, Lewis CE. Plasticity of Macrophage Function During Tumor Progression: Regulation by Distinct Molecular Mechanisms. The Journal of Immunology. 2008;180(4):2011-2017.

[58] Modolell M, Corraliza IM, Link F, Soler G, Eichmann K. Reciprocal Regulation of the Nitric Oxide Synthase/Arginase Balance in Mouse Bone Marrow-Derived Macrophages by Th1 and Th2 Cytokines. European Journal of Immunology. 1995;25(4): 1101-1104.

[59] Rutschman R, Lang R, Hesse M, Ihle JN, Wynn TA, Murray PJ. Cutting Edge: Stat6-Dependent Substrate Depletion Regulates Nitric Oxide Production. The Journal of Immunology. 2001;166(4):2173-2177.

[60] Mylonas KJ, Nair MG, Prieto-Lafuente L, Paape D, Allen JE. Alternatively Activated Macrophages Elicited by Helminth Infection Can Be Reprogrammed to Enable Microbial Killing. The Journal of Immunology. 2009;182(5):3084-3094.

[61] Buttari B, Segoni L, Profumo E, D'Arcangelo D, Rossi S, Facchiano F, Businaro R, Iuliano L, Rigano R. 7-Oxo-Cholesterol Potentiates Pro-Inflammatory Signaling in Human M1 and M2 Macrophages. Biochemical Pharmacology. 2013;86(1):130-137.

[62] Porta C, Rimoldi M, Raes G, Brys L, Ghezzi P, Di Liberto D, Dieli F, Ghisletti S, Natoli G, De Baetselier P, Mantovani A, Sica A. Tolerance and M2 (Alternative) Macrophage Polarization Are Related Processes Orchestrated by P50 Nuclear Factor Kappab. Proceedings of the National Academy of Sciences of the United States of America. 2009;106(35):14978-14983.

[63] Lawrence T, Natoli G. Transcriptional Regulation of Macrophage Polarization: Enabling Diversity with Identity. Nature Reviews Immunology. 2011;11(11):750-761.

[64] Mantovani A, Sica A, Sozzani S, Allavena P, Vecchi A, Locati M. The Chemokine System in Diverse Forms of Macrophage Activation and Polarization. Trends in immunology. 2004;25(12):677-686.

[65] Martinez F, Gordon S, Locati M, Mantovani A. Transcriptional Profiling of the Human Monocyte-to-Macrophage Differentiation and Polarization: New Molecules and Patterns of Gene Expression. The Journal of immunology 2006;177(10):7303-7311.

[66] Hodge S, Matthews G, Mukaro V, Ahern J, Shivam A, Hodge G, Holmes M, Jersmann H, Reynolds PN. Cigarette Smoke-Induced Changes to Alveolar Macrophage

Phenotype and Function Are Improved by Treatment with Procysteine. American Journal of Respiratory Cell and Molecular Biology 2011;44(5):673-681.

[67] Ezekowitz RA, Gordon S. Alterations of Surface Properties by Macrophage Activation: Expression of Receptors for Fc and Mannose-Terminal Glycoproteins and Differentiation Antigens. Contemporary Topics in Immunobiology. 1984;13:33-56.

[68] Doherty TM, Kastelein R, Menon S, Andrade S, Coffman RL. Modulation of Murine Macrophage Function by Il-13. The Journal of Immunology. 1993;151(12):7151-7160.

[69] Doyle AG, Herbein G, Montaner LJ, Minty AJ, Caput D, Ferrara P, Gordon S. Interleukin-13 Alters the Activation State of Murine Macrophages in Vitro: Comparison with Interleukin-4 and Interferon-Gamma. European Journal of Immunology. 1994;24(6):1441-1445.

[70] Murray P, Wynn T. Obstacles and Opportunities for Understanding Macrophage Polarization. Journal of leukocyte biology. 2011;89(4):557-563.

[71] Taylor EL, Megson IL, Haslett C, Rossi AG. Nitric Oxide: A Key Regulator of Myeloid Inflammatory Cell Apoptosis. Cell Death and Differentiation. 2003;10(4):418-430.

[72] Freire-de-Lima CG, Xiao YQ, Gardai SJ, Bratton DL, Schiemann WP, Henson PM. Apoptotic Cells, through Transforming Growth Factor-Beta, Coordinately Induce Anti-Inflammatory and Suppress Pro-Inflammatory Eicosanoid and No Synthesis in Murine Macrophages. The Journal of Biological Chemistry. 2006;281(50):38376-38384.

[73] Beck-Speier I, Karg E, Behrendt H, Stoeger T, Alessandrini F. Ultrafine Particles Affect the Balance of Endogenous Pro-and Anti-Inflammatory Lipid Mediators in the Lung: In-Vitro and in-Vivo Studies. Particle and Fibre Toxicology. 2012;9:27.

[74] Johnston LK, Rims CR, Gill SE, McGuire JK, Manicone AM. Pulmonary Macrophage Subpopulations in the Induction and Resolution of Acute Lung Injury. American Journal of Respiratory Cell and Molecular Biology. 2012;47(4):417-426.

[75] He C, Ryan AJ, Murthy S, Carter AB. Accelerated Development of Pulmonary Fibrosis Via Cu,Zn-Superoxide Dismutase-Induced Alternative Activation of Macrophages. The Journal of Biological Chemistry 2013;288(28):20745-20757.

[76] Tschernig T, Pabst R. What Is the Clinical Relevance of Different Lung Compartments? BMC Pulmonary Medicine 2009;9:39.

[77] Warner AE, Brain JD. The Cell Biology and Pathogenic Role of Pulmonary Intravascular Macrophages. American Journal of Physiology 1990;258(2 Pt 1):L1-12.

[78] Vanderbilt JN, Mager EM, Allen L, Sawa T, Wiener-Kronish J, Gonzalez R, Dobbs LG. Cxc Chemokines and Their Receptors Are Expressed in Type Ii Cells and Upregulated Following Lung Injury. American Journal of Respiratory Cell and Molecular Biology. 2003;29(6):661-668.

[79] Murphy J, Summer R, Wilson AA, Kotton DN, Fine A. The Prolonged Life-Span of Alveolar Macrophages. American Journal of Respiratory Cell and Molecular Biology. 2008;38(4):380-385.

[80] Coleman MM, Ruane D, Moran B, Dunne PJ, Keane J, Mills KH. Alveolar Macrophages Contribute to Respiratory Tolerance by Inducing Foxp3 Expression in Naive T Cells. American Journal of Respiratory Cell and Molecular Biology. 2013;48(6): 773-780.

[81] Mantovani A, Sica A, Locati M. Macrophage Polarization Comes of Age. Immunity. 2005;23(4):344-346.

[82] Jaguin M, Houlbert N, Fardel O, Lecureur V. Polarization Profiles of Human M-Csf-Generated Macrophages and Comparison of M1-Markers in Classically Activated Macrophages from Gm-Csf and M-Csf Origin. Cellular Immunology. 2013;281(1): 51-61.

[83] Ohmori Y, Hamilton TA. Requirement for Stat1 in Lps-Induced Gene Expression in Macrophages. Journal of Leukocyte Biology. 2001;69(4):598-604.

[84] Takeda K, Kamanaka M, Tanaka T, Kishimoto T, Akira S. Impaired Il-13-Mediated Functions of Macrophages in Stat6-Deficient Mice. The Journal of Immunology. 1996;157(8):3220-3222.

[85] Ito S, Ansari P, Sakatsume M, Dickensheets H, Vazquez N, Donnelly RP, Larner AC, Finbloom DS. Interleukin-10 Inhibits Expression of Both Interferon Alpha-and Interferon Gamma-Induced Genes by Suppressing Tyrosine Phosphorylation of Stat1. Blood. 1999;93(5):1456-1463.

[86] Richmond LJ, Alcorn MJ, Pearson C, Cameron G, Thomas T, Eaves CJ, Eaves AC, Holyoake TL. Cml Leukapheresis Products Can Be Enriched for Cd34+Cells and Simultaneously Depleted of Cd15+Cells Using a Simple Ab Cocktail. Cytotherapy. 2002;4(5):407-413.

[87] Watanabe K, Jose PJ, Rankin SM. Eotaxin-2 Generation Is Differentially Regulated by Lipopolysaccharide and Il-4 in Monocytes and Macrophages. The Journal of Immunology. 2002;168(4):1911-1918.

[88] Bonecchi R, Sozzani S, Stine JT, Luini W, D'Amico G, Allavena P, Chantry D, Mantovani A. Divergent Effects of Interleukin-4 and Interferon-Gamma on Macrophage-Derived Chemokine Production: An Amplification Circuit of Polarized T Helper 2 Responses. Blood. 1998;92(8):2668-2671.

[89] Holt PG. Macrophage: Dendritic Cell Interaction in Regulation of the Ige Response in Asthma. Clinical and Experimental Allergy. 1993;23(1):4-6.

[90] Holt PG, Oliver J, Bilyk N, McMenamin C, McMenamin PG, Kraal G, Thepen T. Downregulation of the Antigen Presenting Cell Function(S) of Pulmonary Dendritic

Cells in Vivo by Resident Alveolar Macrophages. Journal of Experimental Medicine. 1993;177(2):397-407.

[91] Strickland D, Kees UR, Holt PG. Regulation of T-Cell Activation in the Lung: Isolated Lung T Cells Exhibit Surface Phenotypic Characteristics of Recent Activation Including Down-Modulated T-Cell Receptors, but Are Locked into the G0/G1 Phase of the Cell Cycle. Immunology. 1996;87(2):242-249.

[92] Wilsher ML, Hughes DA, Haslam PL. Immunoregulatory Properties of Pulmonary Surfactant: Effect of Lung Lining Fluid on Proliferation of Human Blood Lymphocytes. Thorax. 1988;43(5):354-359.

[93] Thepen T, Hoeben K, Breve J, Kraal G. Alveolar Macrophages Down-Regulate Local Pulmonary Immune Responses against Intratracheally Administered T-Cell-Dependent, but Not T-Cell-Independent Antigens. Immunology. 1992;76(1):60-64.

[94] Upham JW, Strickland DH, Bilyk N, Robinson BW, Holt PG. Alveolar Macrophages from Humans and Rodents Selectively Inhibit T-Cell Proliferation but Permit T-Cell Activation and Cytokine Secretion. Immunology. 1995;84(1):142-147.

[95] Holt PG, Kees UR, Shon-Hegrad MA, Rose A, Ford J, Bilyk N, Bowman R, Robinson BW. Limiting-Dilution Analysis of T Cells Extracted from Solid Human Lung Tissue: Comparison of Precursor Frequencies for Proliferative Responses and Lymphokine Production between Lung and Blood T Cells from Individual Donors. Immunology. 1988;64(4):649-654.

[96] Fontenot JD, Gavin MA, Rudensky AY. Foxp3 Programs the Development and Function of Cd4+Cd25+Regulatory T Cells. Nature Immunology 2003;4(4):330-336.

[97] Fontenot JD, Rasmussen JP, Gavin MA, Rudensky AY. A Function for Interleukin 2 in Foxp3-Expressing Regulatory T Cells. Nature Immunology. 2005;6(11):1142-1151.

[98] Mathers C, Loncar D. Projections of Global Mortality and Burden of Disease from 2002 to 2030. PLoS Medicine. 2006;3(11).

[99] Russell RE, Thorley A, Culpitt SV, Dodd S, Donnelly LE, Demattos C, Fitzgerald M, Barnes PJ. Alveolar Macrophage-Mediated Elastolysis: Roles of Matrix Metalloproteinases, Cysteine, and Serine Proteases. American Journal of Physiology Lung Cellular and Molecular Physiology. 2002;283(4):L867-873.

[100] Bracke K, Cataldo D, Maes T, Gueders M, Noel A, Foidart JM, Brusselle G, Pauwels RA. Matrix Metalloproteinase-12 and Cathepsin D Expression in Pulmonary Macrophages and Dendritic Cells of Cigarette Smoke-Exposed Mice. International Archives of Allergy and Immunology. 2005;138(2):169-179.

[101] Mocchegiani E, Giacconi R, Costarelli L. Metalloproteases/Anti-Metalloproteases Imbalance in Chronic Obstructive Pulmonary Disease: Genetic Factors and Treatment Implications. Current Opinion in Pulmonary Medicine. 2011;17 Suppl 1:S11-19.

[102] Finlay GA, O'Driscoll LR, Russell KJ, D'Arcy EM, Masterson JB, FitzGerald MX, O'Connor CM. Matrix Metalloproteinase Expression and Production by Alveolar Macrophages in Emphysema. American Journal of Respiratory and Critical Care Medicine. 1997;156(1):240-247.

[103] Hogg JC, Senior RM. Chronic Obstructive Pulmonary Disease-Part 2: Pathology and Biochemistry of Emphysema. Thorax. 2002;57(9):830-834.

[104] Chapman HA, Riese RJ, Shi GP. Emerging Roles for Cysteine Proteases in Human Biology. Annual Review of Physiology. 1997;59:63-88.

[105] Snider GL. Emphysema: The First Two Centuries--and Beyond. A Historical Overview, with Suggestions for Future Research: Part 1. The American Review of Respiratory Disease. 1992;146(5 Pt 1):1334-1344.

[106] Demedts IK, Morel-Montero A, Lebecque S, Pacheco Y, Cataldo D, Joos GF, Pauwels RA, Brusselle GG. Elevated Mmp-12 Protein Levels in Induced Sputum from Patients with Copd. Thorax. 2006;61(3):196-201.

[107] Chung KF, Adcock IM. Multifaceted Mechanisms in Copd: Inflammation, Immunity, and Tissue Repair and Destruction. The European Respiratory Journal. 2008;31(6): 1334-1356.

[108] Smith JA, Gray AB, Pyne DB, Baker MS, Telford RD, Weidemann MJ. Moderate Exercise Triggers Both Priming and Activation of Neutrophil Subpopulations. The Amercan Journal of Physiology 1996;270(4 Pt 2):R838-R845.

[109] Finkelstein R, Fraser RS, Ghezzo H, Cosio MG. Alveolar Inflammation and Its Relation to Emphysema in Smokers. American Journal of Respiratory and Critical Care Medicine. 1995;152(5 Pt 1):1666-1672.

[110] Jeffery PK. Structural and Inflammatory Changes in Copd: A Comparison with Asthma. Thorax. 1998;53(2):129-136.

[111] Maestrelli P, Paska C, Saetta M, Turato G, Nowicki Y, Monti S, Formichi B, Miniati M, Fabbri LM. Decreased Haem Oxygenase-1 and Increased Inducible Nitric Oxide Synthase in the Lung of Severe Copd Patients. The European Respiratory Journal. 2003;21(6):971-976.

[112] Ichinose M, Sugiura H, Yamagata S, Koarai A, Shirato K. Increase in Reactive Nitrogen Species Production in Chronic Obstructive Pulmonary Disease Airways. American Journal of Respiratory and Critical Care Medicine 2000;162(2 Pt 1):701-706.

[113] Seimetz M, Parajuli N, Pichl A, Veit F, Kwapiszewska G, Weisel FC, Milger K, Egemnazarov B, Turowska A, Fuchs B, Nikam S, Roth M, Sydykov A, Medebach T, Klepetko W, Jaksch P, Dumitrascu R, Garn H, Voswinckel R, Kostin S, Seeger W, Schermuly RT, Grimminger F, Ghofrani HA, Weissmann N. Inducible Nos Inhibition Reverses Tobacco-Smoke-Induced Emphysema and Pulmonary Hypertension in Mice. Cell. 2011;147(2):293-305.

[114] Keatings VM, Collins PD, Scott DM, Barnes PJ. Differences in Interleukin-8 and Tumor Necrosis Factor-Alpha in Induced Sputum from Patients with Chronic Obstructive Pulmonary Disease or Asthma. American Journal of Respiratory and Critical Care Medicine 1996;153(2):530-534.

[115] Bhowmik A, Seemungal TA, Sapsford RJ, Wedzicha JA. Relation of Sputum Inflammatory Markers to Symptoms and Lung Function Changes in Copd Exacerbations. Thorax. 2000;55(2):114-120.

[116] Bucchioni E, Kharitonov SA, Allegra L, Barnes PJ. High Levels of Interleukin-6 in the Exhaled Breath Condensate of Patients with Copd. Respiratory Medicine. 2003;97(12):1299-1302.

[117] Daldegan MB, Teixeira MM, Talvani A. Concentration of Ccl11, Cxcl8 and Tnf-Alpha in Sputum and Plasma of Patients Undergoing Asthma or Chronic Obstructive Pulmonary Disease Exacerbation. Brazilian Journal of Medical and Biological Research. 2005;38(9):1359-1365.

[118] Sapey E, Ahmad A, Bayley D, Newbold P, Snell N, Rugman P, Stockley RA. Imbalances between Interleukin-1 and Tumor Necrosis Factor Agonists and Antagonists in Stable Copd. Journal of Clinical Immunology. 2009;29(4):508-516.

[119] Shaykhiev R, Krause A, Salit J, Strulovici-Barel Y, Harvey B-G, O'Connor T, Crystal R. Smoking-Dependent Reprogramming of Alveolar Macrophage Polarization: Implication for Pathogenesis of Chronic Obstructive Pulmonary Disease. The Journal of immunology. 2009;183(4):2867-2883.

[120] Rosell A, Monso E, Soler N, Torres F, Angrill J, Riise G, Zalacain R, Morera J, Torres A. Microbiologic Determinants of Exacerbation in Chronic Obstructive Pulmonary Disease. Archives of Internal Medicine. 2005;165(8):891-897.

[121] Kunz LI, Lapperre TS, Snoeck-Stroband JB, Budulac SE, Timens W, van Wijngaarden S, Schrumpf JA, Rabe KF, Postma DS, Sterk PJ, Hiemstra PS. Smoking Status and Anti-Inflammatory Macrophages in Bronchoalveolar Lavage and Induced Sputum in Copd. Respiratory Research. 2011;12:34.

[122] Woodruff PG, Koth LL, Yang YH, Rodriguez MW, Favoreto S, Dolganov GM, Paquet AC, Erle DJ. A Distinctive Alveolar Macrophage Activation State Induced by Cigarette Smoking. American Journal of Respiratory and Critical Care Medicine. 2005;172(11):1383-1392.

[123] Churg A, Wang X, Wang RD, Meixner SC, Pryzdial EL, Wright JL. Alpha1-Antitrypsin Suppresses Tnf-Alpha and Mmp-12 Production by Cigarette Smoke-Stimulated Macrophages. American Journal of Respiratory Cell and Molecular Biology. 2007;37(2):144-151.

[124] Ishii T, Abboud RT, Wallace AM, English JC, Coxson HO, Finley RJ, Shumansky K, Pare PD, Sandford AJ. Alveolar Macrophage Proteinase/Antiproteinase Expression and Lung Function/Emphysema. The European Respiratory Journal. 2013.

[125] Pappas K, Papaioannou A, Kostikas K, Tzanakis N. The Role of Macrophages in Obstructive Airways Disease: Chronic Obstructive Pulmonary Disease and Asthma. Cytokine. 2013;64(3):613-625.

[126] Draijer C, Robbe P, Boorsma CE, Hylkema MN, Melgert BN. Characterization of Macrophage Phenotypes in Three Murine Models of House-Dust-Mite-Induced Asthma. Mediators of inflammation. 2013;2013:10.

[127] Bunting MM, Shadie AM, Flesher RP, Nikiforova V, Garthwaite L, Tedla N, Herbert C, Kumar RK. Interleukin-33 Drives Activation of Alveolar Macrophages and Airway Inflammation in a Mouse Model of Acute Exacerbation of Chronic Asthma. BioMed Research International. 2013;2013:250938.

[128] Moon K-A, Kim S, Kim T-B, Yun E, Park C-S, Cho Y, Moon H-B, Lee K-Y. Allergen-Induced Cd11b+Cd11c(Int) Ccr3+Macrophages in the Lung Promote Eosinophilic Airway Inflammation in a Mouse Asthma Model. International Immunology. 2007;19(12):1371-1381.

[129] Heaton T, Rowe J, Turner S, Aalberse R, de Klerk N, Suriyaarachchi D, Serralha M, Holt B, Hollams E, Yerkovich S, Holt K, Sly P, Goldblatt J, Le Souef P, Holt P. An Immunoepidemiological Approach to Asthma: Identification of in-Vitro T-Cell Response Patterns Associated with Different Wheezing Phenotypes in Children. Lancet. 2005;365(9454):142-149.

[130] Kurowska-Stolarska M, Stolarski B, Kewin P, Murphy G, Corrigan CJ, Ying S, Pitman N, Mirchandani A, Rana B, van Rooijen N, Shepherd M, McSharry C, McInnes IB, Xu D, Liew FY. Il-33 Amplifies the Polarization of Alternatively Activated Macrophages That Contribute to Airway Inflammation. The Journal of Immunology. 2009;183(10): 6469-6477.

[131] Simpson J, Gibson P, Yang I, Upham J, James A, Reynolds P, Hodge S, Group ASR. Impaired Macrophage Phagocytosis in Non-Eosinophilic Asthma. Clinical and experimental allergy : journal of the British Society for Allergy and Clinical Immunology. 2013;43(1):29-35.

[132] Gavala ML, Kelly EAB, Esnault S, Kukreja S, Evans MD, Bertics PJ, Chupp GL, Jarjour NN. Segmental Allergen Challenge Enhances Chitinase Activity and Levels of Ccl18 in Mild Atopic Asthma. Clinical and Experimental Allergy. 2013;43(2):187-197.

[133] Siddiqui S, Secor ER, Jr., Silbart LK. Broncho-Alveolar Macrophages Express Chemokines Associated with Leukocyte Migration in a Mouse Model of Asthma. Cellular Immunology. 2013;281(2):159-169.

[134] Lauzon-Joset JF, Marsolais D, Langlois A, Bissonnette EY. Dysregulation of Alveolar Macrophages Unleashes Dendritic Cell-Mediated Mechanisms of Allergic Airway Inflammation. Mucosal immunology. 2013.

[135] Wynn TA. Integrating Mechanisms of Pulmonary Fibrosis. Journal of Experimental Medicine. 2011;208(7):1339-1350.

[136] Sun L, Louie MC, Vannella KM, Wilke CA, LeVine AM, Moore BB, Shanley TP. New Concepts of Il-10-Induced Lung Fibrosis: Fibrocyte Recruitment and M2 Activation in a Ccl2/Ccr2 Axis. American Journal of Physiology Lung Cellular and Molecular Physiology. 2011;300(3):L341-353.

[137] Pechkovsky DV, Prasse A, Kollert F, Engel KM, Dentler J, Luttmann W, Friedrich K, Muller-Quernheim J, Zissel G. Alternatively Activated Alveolar Macrophages in Pulmonary Fibrosis-Mediator Production and Intracellular Signal Transduction. Clinical Immunology. 2010;137(1):89-101.

[138] Mathai SK, Gulati M, Peng X, Russell TR, Shaw AC, Rubinowitz AN, Murray LA, Siner JM, Antin-Ozerkis DE, Montgomery RR, Reilkoff RA, Bucala RJ, Herzog EL. Circulating Monocytes from Systemic Sclerosis Patients with Interstitial Lung Disease Show an Enhanced Profibrotic Phenotype. Laboratory Investigation. 2010;90(6): 812-823.

[139] Wynn TA. Fibrotic Disease and the T(H)1/T(H)2 Paradigm. Nature Reviews Immunology. 2004;4(8):583-594.

[140] Hardie WD, Glasser SW, Hagood JS. Emerging Concepts in the Pathogenesis of Lung Fibrosis. The American Journal of Pathology 2009;175(1):3-16.

[141] Liu T, Jin H, Ullenbruch M, Hu B, Hashimoto N, Moore B, McKenzie A, Lukacs NW, Phan SH. Regulation of Found in Inflammatory Zone 1 Expression in Bleomycin-Induced Lung Fibrosis: Role of Il-4/Il-13 and Mediation Via Stat-6. The Journal of Immunology. 2004;173(5):3425-3431.

[142] Murray LA, Argentieri RL, Farrell FX, Bracht M, Sheng H, Whitaker B, Beck H, Tsui P, Cochlin K, Evanoff HL, Hogaboam CM, Das AM. Hyper-Responsiveness of Ipf/Uip Fibroblasts: Interplay between Tgfbeta1, Il-13 and Ccl2. International Journal of Biochemistry and Cell Biology. 2008;40(10):2174-2182.

[143] Hashimoto S, Gon Y, Takeshita I, Matsumoto K, Maruoka S, Horie T. Transforming Growth Factor-Beta1 Induces Phenotypic Modulation of Human Lung Fibroblasts to Myofibroblast through a C-Jun-Nh2-Terminal Kinase-Dependent Pathway. American Journal of Respiratory and Critical Care Medicine 2001;163(1):152-157.

[144] Migliaccio CT, Buford MC, Jessop F, Holian A. The Il-4ralpha Pathway in Macrophages and Its Potential Role in Silica-Induced Pulmonary Fibrosis. Journal of Leukocyte Biology. 2008;83(3):630-639.

[145] Bargagli E, Margollicci M, Luddi A, Nikiforakis N, Perari MG, Grosso S, Perrone A, Rottoli P. Chitotriosidase Activity in Patients with Interstitial Lung Diseases. Respiratory Medicine. 2007;101(10):2176-2181.

[146] Tercelj M, Salobir B, Simcic S, Wraber B, Zupancic M, Rylander R. Chitotriosidase Activity in Sarcoidosis and Some Other Pulmonary Diseases. Scandinavian Journal of Clinical and Laboratory Investigation. 2009;69(5):575-578.

[147] Everson MP, Chandler DB. Changes in Distribution, Morphology, and Tumor Necrosis Factor-Alpha Secretion of Alveolar Macrophage Subpopulations During the Development of Bleomycin-Induced Pulmonary Fibrosis. The American Journal of Pathology. 1992;140(2):503-512.

[148] Gibbons MA, MacKinnon AC, Ramachandran P, Dhaliwal K, Duffin R, Phythian-Adams AT, van Rooijen N, Haslett C, Howie SE, Simpson AJ, Hirani N, Gauldie J, Iredale JP, Sethi T, Forbes SJ. Ly6chi Monocytes Direct Alternatively Activated Profibrotic Macrophage Regulation of Lung Fibrosis. American Journal of Respiratory and Critical Care Medicine 2011;184(5):569-581.

[149] Cabrera S, Gaxiola M, Arreola JL, Ramirez R, Jara P, D'Armiento J, Richards T, Selman M, Pardo A. Overexpression of Mmp9 in Macrophages Attenuates Pulmonary Fibrosis Induced by Bleomycin. The International Journal of Biochemistry and Cell Biology. 2007;39(12):2324-2338.

[150] Donaldson K, Stone V, Clouter A, Renwick L, MacNee W. Ultrafine Particles. Occupational and Environmental Medicine. 2001;58(3):211-216, 199.

[151] Geiser M, Casaulta M, Kupferschmid B, Schulz H, Semmler-Behnke M, Kreyling W. The Role of Macrophages in the Clearance of Inhaled Ultrafine Titanium Dioxide Particles. American Journal of Respiratory Cell and Molecular Biology. 2008;38(3): 371-376.

[152] Andre E, Stoeger T, Takenaka S, Bahnweg M, Ritter B, Karg E, Lentner B, Reinhard C, Schulz H, Wjst M. Inhalation of Ultrafine Carbon Particles Triggers Biphasic Pro-Inflammatory Response in the Mouse Lung. The European Respiratory Journal. 2006;28(2):275-285.

[153] Stoeger T, Reinhard C, Takenaka S, Schroeppel A, Karg E, Ritter B, Heyder J, Schulz H. Instillation of Six Different Ultrafine Carbon Particles Indicates a Surface Area Threshold Dose for Acute Lung Inflammation in Mice. Environmental Health Perspectives. 2006;114(3):328-333.

[154] Ganguly K, Upadhyay S, Irmler M, Takenaka S, Pukelsheim K, Beckers J, Hamelmann E, Schulz H, Stoeger T. Pathway Focused Protein Profiling Indicates Differential Function for Il-1b,-18 and Vegf During Initiation and Resolution of Lung Inflammation Evoked by Carbon Nanoparticle Exposure in Mice. Particle and Fibre Toxicology 2009;6:31.

[155] Kang CM, Jang AS, Ahn MH, Shin JA, Kim JH, Choi YS, Rhim TY, Park CS. Interleukin-25 and Interleukin-13 Production by Alveolar Macrophages in Response to Particles. American Journal of Respiratory Cell and Molecular Biology. 2005;33(3):290-296.

[156] Takenaka S, Möller W, Semmler-Behnke M, Karg E, Wenk A, Schmid O, Stoeger T, Jennen L, Aichler M, Walch A, Pokhrel S, Mädler L, Eickelberg O, Kreyling W. Efficient Internalization and Intracellular Translocation of Inhaled Gold Nanoparticles in Rat Alveolar Macrophages. Nanomedicine (London, England). 2012;7(6):855-865.

Chapter 3

The Role of MMPs in the Progression of Chronic Lung Inflammatory Diseases

Masaki Fujita

Additional information is available at the end of the chapter

http://dx.doi.org/10.5772/57391

1. Introduction

The alveolar extracellular matrix (ECM) and chronic lung inflammatory diseases, such as pulmonary fibrosis and chronic obstructive pulmonary disease (COPD), are closely connected. Pulmonary fibrosis is associated with ECM production, deposition and remodeling. In contrast, COPD is defined by a loss of the ECM. Matrix metalloproteinases (MMPs) regulate ECM remodeling, and therefore play an important role in the development of chronic lung diseases. MMPs constitute a family of endopeptidases that have a common zinc-based active site. In this chapter, the role of MMPs in pulmonary fibrosis and COPD are discussed, mainly based on the findings in animal models. The effects of MMPs inhibitor on chronic lung disease are also herein discussed.

2. Overview

MMPs constitute a family of endopeptidases with a zinc molecule in their active site and a dependency on Ca^{2+} for their activity. MMPs are thought to be responsible for the turnover and degradation of the ECM [1-3]. In the lungs, these proteinases are synthesized and secreted by diverse cell types, including mesenchymal cells, macrophages, polymorphonuclear cells, alveolar type II epithelial cells, fibroblasts, smooth muscle cells, the lung parenchyma and inflammatory cells [4].

Classification

The most commonly used classifications are based partly on the historical assessment of the substrate specificity of the MMPs, and partly on the cellular localization of the MMPs. They can be divided into two main groups based on their domain and compartment location: basic secreted MMPs (collagenases, gelatinases and stromelysins) and membrane-anchored (the membrane-type) MMPs (MT-MMPs). The collagenases are capable of degrading triple-helical fibrillar collagens into distinct 3/4 and 1/4 fragments. These collagens are the major components of bone, cartilage and dentin, and MMPs are the only known mammalian enzymes capable of degrading them. The collagenases are MMP-1, -8, -13 and -18. In addition, MMP-14 has also been shown to cleave fibrillar collagen, and there is evidence that MMP-2 is capable of collagenolysis. The main substrates of the gelatinases are type IV collagen and gelatin, and these enzymes are distinguished by the presence of an additional domain inserted into the catalytic domain. This gelatin-binding region is positioned immediately before the zinc-binding motif, and forms a separate folding unit that does not disrupt the structure of the catalytic domain. The gelatinases are MMP-2 and MMP-9. The stromelysins display a broad ability to cleave extracellular matrix proteins, but are unable to cleave the triple-helical fibrillar collagens. The three canonical members of this group are MMP-3, -10, and -11. All six membrane-type MMPs (MMP14, -15, -16, -17, -24, and -25) have a furin cleavage site in the pro-peptide, which is a feature also shared by MMP-11. There are a number of MMPs that do not fit into any of the traditional groups, such as matrilysins (MMP-7, MMP-26). In addition, MMP-19, enamelysin (MMP-20), MMP-21, MMP-23A and 23B, MMP-27 and epilysin (MMP-28) have recently been reported and are still being characterized (Summarized in Table 1).

Structure

To be classified as an MMP, a protein needs to have at least the conserved pro-domain and catalytic domain (Figure 1). The pro-domain of a typical MMP is 80 amino acids, and contains the consensus sequence, PRCXXPD. The exception is MMP23, in which the crucial cysteine residue is found in a distinct amino acid sequence. The catalytic domain of a typical MMP contains a zinc ion (Zn^{2+}) in the active site that is ligated to three conserved histidine residues in the sequence HEXXHXXGXXH. The glutamic acid residue (E) in this catalytic motif provides the nucleophile that severs peptide bonds. The backbone structures of the MMP catalytic domain, include a characteristic Met turn on the carboxy side of the zinc active site, so matrix metalloproteinases have a methionine residue that is always conserved. This residue is part of a 1,4-β-turn that loops the polypeptide chain beneath the catalytic zinc ion and forms a hydrophobic base for the zinc-binding site. This is caused by a conserved methionine residue downstream of the zinc-binding site, which is similar to those of the astacin-, reprolysin- (also known as a disintegrin and metalloproteinase (ADAMs)) and serralysin-family metalloproteinases.

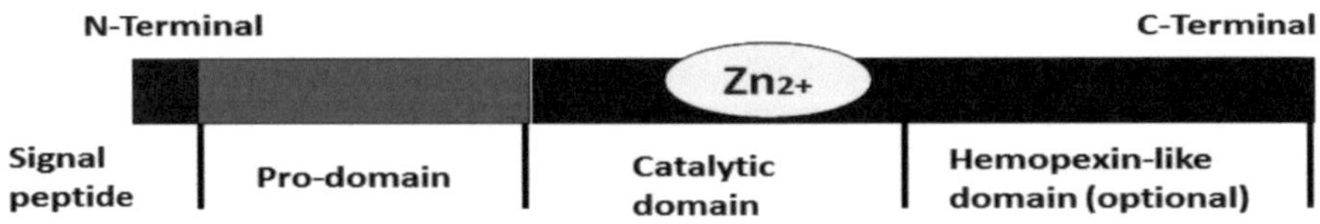

Figure 1. The structure of the MMPs

Group name	Number	Substrates
Collagenase-1	MMP-1	Collagen I, II, III, X, Casein
Gelatinase-A	MMP-2	CCL7, CXCL12, Collagens IV, V, VII, XI, Gelatin, Fibronectin
Stromelysin-1	MMP-3	E-cadherin, Laminin, Latent TGF-beta, Collagens III, IV, VII, IX, Casein, Fibronectin
Matrilysin	MMP-7	Pro-alpha-defensins, Fas L, Latent TNF, Syndecan-1, E-cadherin, Elastin, Collagens IV, Casein, Fibronectin
Collagenase-2	MMP-8	CXCL5, Collagens I, II, III, Casein
Gelatinase-B	MMP-9	Zona occludens 1, alpha1-antiproteinase, Latent TGF-beta, Latent VEGF, Fibrin, NG2 proteoglycan, Collagens III, IV, V, Gelatin
Stromelysin-2	MMP-10	Collagens III, IV, V, Casein, Fibronectin
Stromelysin-3	MMP-11	Fibronectin
Metalloelastase	MMP-12	Latent TNF, Elastin, Gelatin, Casein
Collagenase-3	MMP-13	Type I, II fibrillar collagen
MT1-MMP	MMP-14	ProMMP2, Fibrillar collagens, Fibrin, Syndecan-1, laminin
MT2-MMP	MMP-15	Fibrin
MT3-MMP	MMP-16	Fibrin, Syndecan-1
MT4-MMP	MMP-17	ND
MMP-19	MMP-19	ND
Enamelysin	MMP-20	Amelogenin
MMP-21	MMP-21	ND
MMP-23A	MMP-23A	ND
MMP-23B	MMP-23B	ND
MT5-MMP	MMP-24	ND
MT6-MMP	MMP-25	ND
Matrilysin-2	MMP-26	ND
MMP-27	MMP-27	ND
Epilysin	MMP-28	ND

ND=Not determined.

Table 1. A list of the currently known MMPs

Several MMPs have the hemopexin-like C-terminal domain, which is linked to the catalytic domain by a flexible hinge region. The minimum domain structure is characteristic of matrilysins (MMP-7 and MMP-26). Stromelysin (MMP-3 and MMP-10), collagenases (MMP-1, 8,

13), MMP-12, enamelysin (MMP-20) and MMP-27 have several hemopexin domains. A similar domain structure is present in MMP-11, MMP-28 and MMP-21, which have a furin-like target sequence inserted in their pro-domains. Membrane-type MMPs have membrane-anchored modules of glycosylphophatidylinositol, which form type I or type II transmembrane segments. MMP-23A and 23B have an immunoglobulin-like domain. MMP-2 and MMP-9 are secreted MMPs with gelatinolytic activity, and are characterized by the presence of fibronectin type II modules [1-3].

Regulation

The activation of MMPs can be mediated by other MMPs or proteases, and some are activated intracellularly by furins. In addition, various chemicals, such as organomercurials, urea, some detergents and reactive oxygen species, can act as activators of MMPs. Although the healthy adult lung is not a major source of MMPs, parenchymal cells, such as the airway epithelium, fibroblasts and smooth muscle have the capacity to express active MMPs following stimulation by a variety of agents, such as infectious pathogens, environmental toxins, growth factors and cytokines.

Since MMPs may cause significant host damage, they are tightly regulated. MMPs are regulated at four main levels: gene transcription, proenzyme activation, activity inhibition and compartmentalization. First, they are rarely stored, and require gene transcription before secretion, the exception being neutrophil MMP-8 and -9. Second, MMPs are either secreted as pro-enzymes that require proteolytic cleavage, or in the case of MT-MMPs, are activated intracellularly by pro-protein convertases, such as furin. This processing exposes the catalytic cleft, a mechanism known as the cysteine switch [5]. Third, specific inhibitors of MMPs, the tissue inhibitors of metalloproteinases (TIMPs), are secreted proteins that bind MMPs in a 1:1 manner to prevent their enzymatic activity [6]. TIMPs comprise a family of four protease inhibitors (TIMPs 1-4). The balance of MMPs to TIMPs therefore determines the matrix turnover, where either an excess of MMPs or a deficit of TIMPs may result in excess ECM degradation. The major endogenous MMP inhibitor in serum is α2-macroglobulin, which binds MMPs and leads to their clearance by endocytosis. Finally, MMPs can be compartmentalized in close proximity to the cell.

Synthetic MMP inhibitors and clinical implications

A number of rationally-designed MMP inhibitors have shown some promise in the treatment of pathologies in which MMPs have been implicated. Two major approaches were undertaken to counterbalance such MMP activity: substrate peptide mimics and small synthetic molecules.

Macpherson and colleagues developed a nonpeptidic hydroxamic acid inhibitor (CGS 27023A) of the stromelysin group of MMPs, which was orally bioactive and blocked the erosion of cartilage matrix in an *in vivo* rabbit model of cartilage degradation [7]. Batimastat, a broad spectrum MMP inhibitor, showed prolonged survival in an animal model of cancer and some efficacy in phase I clinical trials, but its development was hindered by its low bioavailability and limited solubility [8]. Marimastat, a low-molecular-weight substrate peptide-based hydroximate (inhibitor of MMPs -1, -8, and -13), and prinomastat, based on a sulphonamide-hydroximate scaffold (inhibitor of MMPs -2, -3, and -13), failed during phase III clinical trials for cancer treatment [9]. In addition, cipemastat (Ro 32-3555), an MMP-1-selective inhibitor, demonstrated limited efficacy in clinical trials. The development of several other MMP inhibitors was stopped due to their systemic toxicity, a lack of any correlation between the activity of MMP inhibitors and the MMP levels in the plasma and poor efficacy [10].

Doxycycline, at sub-antimicrobial doses, inhibits MMP activity, and has been used in various experimental systems for this purpose, such as for recalcitrant recurrent corneal erosions. It is used clinically for the treatment of periodontal disease, and is the only MMP inhibitor that is widely available clinically. Minocycline, another tetracycline antibiotic, has also been shown to inhibit MMP activity. For example, tetracyclines, which are used in the treatment of arthritis, have been shown to reduce the activity of MMPs -1, -2 and -9 [11].

3. The inflammatory process

The main activity of MMPs is considered to be the degradation of the ECM. However, matrix degradation is neither the sole function, nor the main function, of these proteinases. Recent findings indicate that MMPs play an important role in the regulation of cytokine and chemokine release and activation, which are key steps in the immune response [2, 3, 12-14]. For example, MMP-1,-2, -3, -7, -9, and -12 are able to process pro-tumor-necrosis factor (TNF)-α into soluble active TNF-α. MMP-2, -3 and -9 also have the ability to cleave interleukin (IL)-1β, generating a more active form. MMP-9 controls the IL-2-dependent proliferation of T lymphocytes. MMP-8, -13 and -14 can cleave IL-8 to generate truncated forms with increased activity. Therefore, inflammatory cytokines and MMPs are interconnected.

An essential pro-inflammatory mediator that is regulated by metalloproteinase activity is TNF, which is produced as a 26-kDa membrane-associated protein (proTNF) that is cleaved by TNF-converting enzyme (TACE) into a soluble 17.5-kDa cytokine. Because synthetic metalloproteinase inhibitors block this cleavage, it was suggested that TACE was an MMP. However, when the convertase activity was purified and cloned, TACE was found to be identical to ADAM17 [15, 16]. The cleavage of proTNF by ADAM17 is specific [17]. Since the release of active TNF is reduced by 90% in cells derived from ADAM17-deficient mice, ADAM17 seems to be the principal physiological TNF-converting enzyme *in vivo*. Several MMPs (including MMP-1, -2, -3, -9 and -17) can process proTNF to its active form *in vitro* [18, 19]. MMP-7 and MMP-12 also activate proTNF in macrophages. The high-level release of TNF in response to bacteria and toxic shock by MMP-7 and MMP-12 processing might elicit the constitutive release of TNF from macrophages that is required for common functions, such as tissue resorption and resolution, in response to injury.

Similarly, IL-1, a potent pro-inflammatory cytokine, requires proteolytic processing for activation, a process attributed to the IL-1-converting enzyme (ICE, caspase-1). Although the function of ICE had been well established *in vitro*, studies using ICE-deficient mice provided evidence of other mechanisms of IL-1 activation [20]. It was subsequently discovered that MMP-2, -3 and -9 can cleave and activate the IL-1 precursor [21]. Furthermore, after activating IL-1, MMP-3 degrades the biologically active cytokine [21], which can also be inactivated *in vitro* by MMP-1, -2 and -9 [22]. These data indicate a dual role for MMPs in the biphasic modulation of inflammatory-mediator activity. MMPs are involved in both the activation and inactivation of these inflammatory molecules.

Moreover, several studies have indicated that MMPs can either directly or indirectly affect the activity interferon-γ [23], vascular endothelial growth factor [24], epidermal growth factors [25], fibroblast growth factors [26] and transforming growth factor (TGF)-β. As shown using TGF-β-deficient mice, this cytokine functions to restrain mononuclear inflammation [27-29]. In both cells and tissue-explant models, MMP-3 [30], MMP-9 [31] and MMP-14 [32] have been shown or suggested to activate a proportion of the total TGF-β.

Lopez-Boado et al. reported a 25-fold induction of MMP-7 in lung epithelial cells following infection with *Escherichia coli* [33] and *Pseudomonas aeruginosa*, [34] which could explain the upregulation of this enzyme in the airway of cystic fibrosis patients who are commonly infected with these bacteria. It has also been shown that proinflammatory cytokines, such as IL-1β and TNF-α, upregulate the expression of MMP-9 in human airway epithelial cells following a one-day treatment [35].

4. Pulmonary fibrosis and MMPs

Lung inflammation is deeply associated with the process of pulmonary fibrosis. MMP-9 was observed in alveolar macrophages from idiopathic pulmonary fibrosis patients [36] and in the bronchoalveolar lavage (BAL) fluid from patients with bleomycin-induced pulmonary fibrosis [37, 38]. An mRNA study also supported that the activation of MMP-2 and MMP-9, both gelatinases, is involved in pulmonary fibrosis [39]. The function of other MMPs, such as collagenases or stromelysins, in pulmonary fibrosis is still unclear, despite their importance in ECM deposition. Edwards and colleagues reported that mast cells harvested from the tissues of patients with interstitial lung diseases demonstrated the expression of MMP-1. MMP-1 has thus been reported to be important for controlling fibrogenesis in humans [40]. Although the existence of MMP-1 is unclear in rodents [41], other collagenases, such as MMP-13, have been detected [42]. Similarly, collagenase activity has been observed after bleomycin administration [37]. An immunohistochemical analysis demonstrated that MMP-13 expression was present after bleomycin administration [43]. However, other researchers have reported that the MMP-9 (gelatinase B), MMP-3 (stromelysin-1) and interstitial collagenase gene expression did not significantly change after bleomycin administration [44].

5. Therapeutic trials for pulmonary fibrosis

As mentioned previously, doxycycline inhibits MMP activity. We demonstrated that the early administration of doxycycline inhibited early inflammation and resulted in an inhibition of the development of pulmonary fibrosis through the inhibition of early inflammation [45]. However, doxycycline did not affect established pulmonary fibrosis. A MMPs inhibitor, batimastat, was reported to attenuate pulmonary fibrosis in mice [38]. Batimastat inhibited both MMP-2 and TIMP-1, and resulted in the attenuation of pulmonary fibrosis. In contrast, a MMPs inhibitor, CGS27023A, blocked the anti-fibrotic MMPs and resulted in an augmentation of the ECM [43].

MMPs play an important role in the development of pulmonary fibrosis. However, there are conflicting hypotheses regarding whether MMPs have anti-fibrotic properties [46]. Researchers should focus on when and what type of MMPs inhibitor(s) should be used for pulmonary fibrosis.

6. COPD and MMPs

Both alveolar and bronchial inflammation have been shown to be present in human COPD. Hence, chronic inflammation contributes to the development of COPD through the destruction of alveoli and the induction of MMPs. Recently, the role of MMPs has been given increasing attention as a possible mechanism underlying the development of pulmonary emphysema. Additionally, the inflammatory cells invading the lung during the course of COPD are also a major source of different MMPs. It has been shown that neutrophils and macrophages are the predominant inflammatory cells in the lungs of COPD patients [47, 48].

Lipopolysaccharide (LPS) is a strong proinflammatory compound present in the cell wall of gram-negative bacteria. Acute LPS instillation induces apoptotic cell death in bronchial epithelial cells at early time points, and neutrophil apoptosis in the lungs at later time points [49, 50], and this is associated with the production of MMPs, mainly gelatinase [51]. LPS leads to the recruitment of neutrophils and macrophage activation with concomitant airspace enlargement [52, 53]. Although humans tolerate bacterial pneumonia without any residual emphysema, the chronic instillation of LPS was found to induce COPD-like changes. Bacterial endotoxin was demonstrated to be present in high concentrations in tobacco (approximately 20 μg/cigarette), and bioactive LPS could be detected in both mainstream and sidestream cigarette smoke (approximately 0.12-0.2 μg/cigarette) [54, 55]. Repetitive LPS instillation for 12 weeks led to COPD-like changes [56]. This mouse model mimicked several important pathological changes that are observed in COPD patients. These mice demonstrated goblet cell metaplasia in the larger airways, thickening of the airway walls and irreversible alveolar enlargements [57]. It is well known that LPS induces TNF-α. TNF-α overexpression in mice has been reported to have diverse effects, including the induction of pulmonary emphysema and pulmonary fibrosis. At first, the overexpression of TNF-α in the lungs of mice was thought to lead to pulmonary fibrosis [58, 59]. In contrast, TNF-α overexpressing mice bred in Denver demonstrated pulmonary emphysema [60]. Chronic inflammation, a reduced elastic recoil, a huge lung size and an activation of MMPs (mainly MMP-2 and MMP-9) were all observed in these mice, along with a progression of pulmonary hypertension [61]. In addition, this mouse model was insensitive to fibrogenesis factor, bleomycin and TGF-β [62]. Many evidence have demonstrated that TNF-α plays a critical role in smoking-related emphysema [63]. Taking these findings into consideration, TNF-α is considered to play a crucial role in the development of COPD and MMPs, mainly MMP-2 and MMP-9 is associated with the COPD pathogenesis.

Several transgenic mouse strains with targeted expression of cytokines show COPD-like lesions, such as airspace enlargement, thickening of the airway walls and subepithelial fibrosis without any exposure to a specific agent [64, 65]. An overexpression of IL-13 in the murine lung caused an asthma-like eosinophil- and lymphocyte-rich inflammation, goblet cell hyperplasia, airway fibrosis and alveolar enlargement [66, 67]. The induced overexpression of interferon (IFN)-γ in the lungs of mice caused a phenotype mimicking human COPD [68]. In these models, the overexpression of these inflammatory cytokines was associated with an increased expression of MMPs (mainly gelatinase) and cysteine proteases, including cathepsins. Similarly, macrophage colony stimulating factor (M-CSF)-deficient mice, surfactant protein D (SP-D)-deficient mice and integrin αvβ6-deficient mice also develop air space enlargement [69-71]. The macrophages of SP-D-deficient mice have increased oxidant production, which activates nuclear factor (NF)-κB and subsequently leads to MMP expression [72]. NF-kB is also well known to be a transcription factor involved in the induction of TNF-α. Inflammation and MMPs activation (mainly gelatinase) contribute to the development of COPD.

Another mechanism for COPD involves macrophage elastase (MMP-12). MMP-12 is nearly undetectable in healthy macrophages, while MMP-12 is expressed in the alveolar macrophages of human cigarette smokers. Of note, MMP-12 knockout mice did not develop emphysema in response to long-term cigarette smoke exposure [73, 74]. MMP-12 knockout mice also failed to recruit macrophages into their lungs in response to cigarette smoke. Neutrophil elastase-deficient mice were significantly protected from the development of pulmonary emphysema after cigarette smoke exposure [75]. Mice that constitutively overexpress human MMP-1 develop spontaneous air space enlargement, showing that MMP-1 can drive pulmonary destruction [76]. Since that report, numerous transgenic mouse models have been developed, in which emphysema-like changes are induced. The absence of MMP inhibitors can also result in abnormal pulmonary matrix turnover, as TIMP-3 deficient mice spontaneously develop air space enlargement at two weeks of age [77].

The functional importance of MMP activity in these models was confirmed by crossing emphysema-developing mice with MMP-knockout mice. For example, in the IL-13 overexpression model, a deficiency of MMP-9 or MMP-12 results in reduced pathological changes and less respiratory failure [78]. Similarly, crossing integrin αvβ6-deficient mice with MMP-12-deficient mice prevents the development of age-related emphysema [79].

MMPs seem to be strongly related to the development of COPD [80]. In a clinical study, there were increases in the pulmonary expression of MMP -1 [81], MMP-2 [82], MMP-8 [83], MMP -9 [84], MMP-12 [85] and MMP-14[82] in COPD patients. For example, Finlay and colleagues detected collagenase activity in BAL fluid samples from 100% of emphysematous patients but in only 10% of smoking controls; and MMP-9 was present in 60% of patients compared to 20% in the control group [84]. Segura-Valdez and colleagues showed a significant upregulation of MMPs -1, -2, -8, and -9 in the BAL fluid samples obtained from COPD patients [86]. In another study, Imai and colleagues reported the detection of MMP-1 mRNA by *in situ* hybridization, and also found protein expression and enzymatic activity in the lung samples of patients with emphysema. However, there was no MMP-1 detected in the lungs of normal control subjects [81]. Additionally, Ohnishi and colleagues documented a more than three-fold increase in the level of MMP-2 protein and activation in lung samples from emphysematous patients compared to subjects in the control group [82]. Another study reported an increase in the MMP-9 protein level in 40% of COPD patients compared to healthy subjects. The location of the MMP-9 expression was confirmed by an immunohistochemical analysis to be in the bronchial epithelium and submucosal areas [87]. Furthermore, an extracellular MMP inducer, called basigin, a member of the immunoglobulin G (IgG) superfamily, were increased in smokers' BAL fluid samples [88]. The extracellular MMP inducer was prominent in the bronchial glands, bronchial epithelium and alveolar macrophages. An increase in the level of MMP-9 has also been reported in the sputum of patients with chronic bronchitis compared to control subjects [89].

MMP-9 and MMP-12 play key roles in the development of COPD in mice. However, studies in patients suggest that the spectrum of MMPs in human disease may differ significantly from these models. Studies of MMP activity demonstrate divergent results at different stages of disease evolution, and lead to controversy about which MMPs are critical in pulmonary disease in humans. Taking the data from both clinical and animal studies into consideration, MMP-9 is the most compelling molecule related to the development of COPD. In contrast, MMP-12 is essential for the cigarette smoke-induced pathology in the mouse, but may not be equally critical in human disease.

7. Therapeutic trials for COPD

MMP inhibition could be a promising candidate therapy for COPD. In fact, a MMP inhibitor, GM6001, has been reported to block the emphysematous changes associated with methyl-prednisolone-induced emphysema in rats [90]. However, past experiences, including our own study, have shown that a broad spectrum MMP inhibitor would be of limited benefit [91-93]. In fact, our preliminary study using CGS27023A, an MMP inhibitor, or doxycycline, did not improve the COPD in mice with TNF-α overexpression (unpublished data). Nonselective MMP inhibitors, such as marimastat, have major side effects. Isoenzyme-selective inhibitors or inhaled delivery may be needed. A dual MMP9–MMP12 inhibitor (AZ11557272) was shown to prevent emphysema, small airway fibrosis and inflammation in guinea pigs that were exposed to cigarette smoke over a six-month period [94], but its clinical development has now been stopped for some unknown reason. MMP-9 is potentially a good target for patients with emphysema, but progress in the development of drugs targeting MMP-9 has been disappointing, because it has proved to be difficult to discover safe and selective MMP-9 inhibitors [93]. A more sophisticated approach is therefore required in the future.

8. Conclusion

There is a controversy concerning the role of MMPs in the development of chronic inflammatory lung diseases. There were two possible but conflicting roles of MMPs: promoting the deposition of the ECM by facilitating fibroblast migration, or degenerating the ECM. MMPs play important roles in the degradation of the ECM and recovery from lung damage. Similar to inflammation, MMPs activation was observed in both pulmonary fibrosis and COPD. The role of MMPs in inflammatory lung diseases is therefore complex. The different MMPs show variations in terms of their effecting depending on different condition. In addition, MMP inhibitors appear to work in different ways. More precise and specific studies of both the proteins themselves and their specific inhibitors will be needed in the future. Moreover, there are discrepancies between mice and humans. Novel therapeutic agents targeting MMPs for use against chronic inflammation are currently under development, and more will likely be developed as more is learned about the MMPs and their functions. This information is summarized in Figure 2.

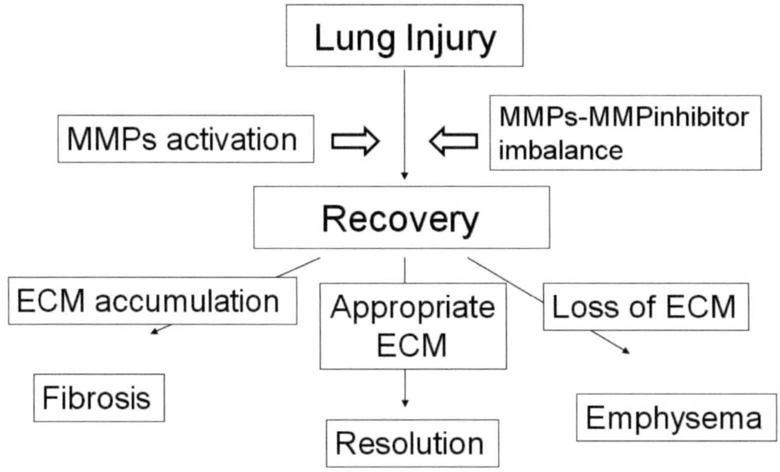

Figure 2. A schematic drawing of the relationship between MMPs and lung injury.

Abbreviations

a disintegrin and metalloproteinase (ADAMs)

bronchoalveolar lavage (BAL)

chronic obstructive pulmonary disease (COPD)

extracellular matrix (ECM)

IL-1-converting enzyme (ICE)

immunoglobulin G (IgG)

interleukin (IL)

interferon (IFN)

lipopolysaccharide (LPS)

macrophage colony stimulating factor (M-CSF)

matrix metalloproteinases (MMPs)

membrane-type MMPs (MT-MMPs)

nuclear factor (NF)

surfactant protein D (SP-D)

tissue inhibitors of metalloproteinases (TIMPs)

tumor-necrosis factor (TNF)

TNF-converting enzyme (TACE)

transforming growth factor (TGF)

Author details

Masaki Fujita*

Address all correspondence to: mfujita@fukuoka-u.ac.jp

Department of Respiratory Medicine, Fukuoka University Hospital, Fukuoka, Japan

References

[1] Clark IM Edit. Matrix metalloproteinase protocols, second edition. Humana Press/ Springer: New York; 2010

[2] William C. Parks, Carole L. Wilson & Yolanda S. López-Boado. Matrix metalloproteinases as modulators of inflammation and innate immunity. Nature Reviews Immunology 2006;4: 617-629

[3] Lydia Sorokin. The impact of the extracellular matrix on inflammation.Nature Reviews Immunology 2010;10: 712-723

[4] O'Connor CM, FitzGerald MX. Matrix metalloproteases and lung disease. Thorax 1994;49: 602-609.

[5] Van Wart HE, Birkedal-Hansen H. The cysteine switch: a principle of regulation of metalloproteinase activity with potential applicability to the entire matrix metalloproteinase gene family. Proc Natl Acad Sci USA 1990;87: 5578–5582.

[6] Brew K, Dinakarpandian D, Nagase H. Tissue inhibitors of metalloproteinases: evolution, structure and function. Biochim Biophys Acta 2000;1477: 267–283.

[7] MacPherson LJ, Bayburt EK, Capparelli MP, et al. Discovery of CGS 27023A, a non-peptidic, potent, and orally active stromelysin inhibitor that blocks cartilage degradation in rabbits. J Med Chem 1997;40: 2525-2532.

[8] Coussens LM, Fingleton B, Matrisian LM. Matrix metalloproteinase inhibitors and cancer: trials and tribulations. Science 2002;295: 2387-2392

[9] Broker LE, Giaccone G. The role of new agents in the treatment of non-small cell lung cancer. Eur J Cancer 2002;38: 2347-2361

[10] Hoekstra R, Eskens FA, Verweij J. Matrix metalloproteinase inhibitors: current developments and future perspectives. Oncologist 2001;6: 415-427

[11] Whelan, CJ. Metalloprotease inhibitors as anti-inflammatory agents: an evolving target? Curr Opin Investig Drugs 2004;5: 511-516

[12] Morrison CJ, Butler GS, Rodriguez D, Overall CM. Matrix metalloproteinase proteomics: substrates, targets, and therapy. Curr Opin Cell Biol 2009;21: 645–653.

[13] Cauwe B, Van den Steen PE, Opdenakker G. The biochemical, biological, and pathological kaleidoscope of cell surface substrates processed by matrix metalloproteinases. Crit Rev Biochem Mol Biol 2007;42: 113–185.

[14] Struyf S, Proost P, Van Damme J. Regulation of the immune response by the interaction of chemokines and proteases. Adv Immunol 2003;81: 1–44.

[15] ack RA, Rauch CT, Kozlosky CJ, Peschon JJ, Slack JL, Wolfson MF, Castner BJ, Stocking KL, Reddy P, Srinivasan S, Nelson N, Boiani N, Schooley KA, Gerhart M, Davis R, Fitzner JN, Johnson RS, Paxton RJ, March CJ, Cerretti DP. A metalloproteinase disintegrin that releases tumour-necrosis factor-α from cells. Nature 1997;385:729–733.

[16] Moss ML, Jin SL, Milla ME, Bickett DM, Burkhart W, Carter HL, Chen WJ, Clay WC, Didsbury JR, Hassler D, Hoffman CR, Kost TA, Lambert MH, Leesnitzer MA, McCauley P, McGeehan G, Mitchell J, Moyer M, Pahel G, Rocque W, Overton LK, Schoenen F, Seaton T, Su JL, Warner J, Willarad D, Becherer JD. Cloning of a disintegrin metalloproteinase that processes precursor tumour-necrosis factor-α. Nature 1997;385:733–736.

[17] Mohan MJ, Seaton T, Mitchell J, Howe A, Blackburn K, Burkhart W, Moyer M, Patel I, Waitt GM, Becherer JD, Moss ML, Milla ME. The tumor necrosis factor-α converting enzyme (TACE): a unique metalloproteinase with highly defined substrate selectivity. Biochemistry 2002;41:9462–9469.

[18] English WR, Puente XS, Freije JM, Knauper V, Amour A, Merryweather A, Lopez-Otin C, Murphy G. Membrane type 4 matrix metalloproteinase (MMP17) has tumor necrosis factor-α convertase activity but does not activate pro-MMP2. J Biol Chem 2000;275: 14046–14055.

[19] Visse R, Nagase H. Matrix metalloproteinases and tissue inhibitors of metalloproteinases: structure, function, and biochemistry. Circ Res 2003; 92: 827–839.

[20] Fantuzzi G, Ku G, Harding MW, Livingston DJ, Sipe JD, Kuida K, Flavell RA, Dinarello CA. Response to local inflammation of IL-1β-converting enzyme-deficient mice. J Immunol 1997;158: 1818–1824.

[21] Schönbeck U, Mach F, Libby P. Generation of biologically active IL-1β by matrix metalloproteinases: a novel caspase-1-independent pathway of IL-1β processing. J Immunol 1998;161: 3340–3346.

[22] Ito A, Mukaiyama A, Itoh Y, Nagase H, Thogersen IB, Enghild JJ, Sasaguri Y, Mori Y. Degradation of interleukin 1β by matrix metalloproteinases. J Biol Chem 1996; 271: 14657–14660.

[23] Nelissen I, Martens E, Van den Steen PE, Proost P, Ronsse I, Opdenakker G. Gelatinase B/matrix metalloproteinase-9 cleaves interferon-β and is a target for immunotherapy. Brain 2003;126:1371–1381.

[24] Bergers G, Brekken R, McMahon G, Vu TH, Itoh T, Tamaki K, Tanzawa K, Thorpe P, Itohara S, Werb Z, Hanahan D. Matrix metalloproteinase-9 triggers the angiogenic switch during carcinogenesis. Nature Cell Biol 2000; 2: 737–744.

[25] Suzuki M, Raab G, Moses MA, Fernandez CA, Klagsbrun M. Matrix metalloproteinase-3 releases active heparin-binding EGF-like growth factor by cleavage at a specific juxtamembrane site. J Biol Chem 1997; 272:31730–31737.

[26] Levi E, Fridman R, Miao HQ, Ma YS, Yayon A, Vlodavsky I. Matrix metalloproteinase 2 releases active soluble ectodomain of fibroblast growth factor receptor 1. Proc Natl Acad Sci USA 1996;93:7069–7074.

[27] Shull MM, Ormsby I, Kier AB, Pawlowski S, Diebold RJ, Yin M, Allen R, Sidman C, Proetzel G, Calvin D, Annunziata N, Doetschman T. Targeted disruption of the mouse transforming growth factor-β 1 gene results in multifocal inflammatory disease. Nature 1992;359: 693–699.

[28] Kulkarni AB, Karlsson S. Transforming growth factor-β 1 knockout mice. A mutation in one cytokine gene causes a dramatic inflammatory disease. Am J Pathol 1993;143: 3–9.

[29] Munger JS, Huang X, Kawakatsu H, Griffiths MJ, Dalton SL, Wu J, Pittet JF, Kaminski N, Garat C, Matthay MA, Rifkin DB, Sheppard D. The integrin αvβ6 binds and activates latent TGFβ1: a mechanism for regulating pulmonary inflammation and fibrosis. Cell 1999;96: 319–328.

[30] Maeda S, Dean DD, Gomez R, Schwartz Z, Boyan BD. The first stage of transforming growth factor β1 activation is release of the large latent complex from the extracellular matrix of growth plate chondrocytes by matrix vesicle stromelysin-1 (MMP-3). Calcif Tissue Int 2002;70: 54–65.

[31] Yu Q, Stamenkovic I. Cell surface-localized matrix metalloproteinase-9 proteolytically activates TGF-β and promotes tumor invasion and angiogenesis. Genes Dev 2000;14: 163–176.

[32] Karsdal MA, Larsen L, Engsig MT, Lou H, Ferreras M, Lochter A, Delaissé JM, Foged NT. Matrix metalloproteinase-dependent activation of latent transforming growth factor-β controls the conversion of osteoblasts into osteocytes by blocking osteoblast apoptosis. J Biol Chem 2002;277: 44061–44067.

[33] López-Boado YS, Wilson CL, Hooper LV, Gordon JI, Hultgren SJ, Parks WC. Bacterial exposure induces and activates matrilysin in mucosal epithelial cells. J Cell Biol 2000;148: 1305-1315.

[34] Lopez-Boado YS, Wilson CL, Parks WC. Regulation of matrilysin expression in airway epithelial cells by Pseudomonas aeruginosa flagellin. J Biol Chem 2001;276: 41417-41423.

[35] Yao PM, Delclaux C, d'Ortho MP, Maitre B, Harf A, Lafuma C. Cell-matrix interactions modulate 92-kD gelatinase expression by human bronchial epithelial cells. Am J Respir Cell Mol Biol 1998;18: 813-822.

[36] Lemjabbar H, Gosset P, Lechapt-Zalcman E, Franco-Montoya ML, Wallaert B, Harf A, Lafuma C. Overexpression of alveolar macrophage gelatinase B (MMP-9) in patients with idiopathic pulmonary fibrosis. Effect of steroid and immunosuppressive treatment. Am J Respir Cell Mol Biol 1999;20: 903-913.

[37] Bakowska J, Adamson IY. Collagenase and gelatinase activities in bronchoalveolar lavage fluids during bleomycin-induced lung injury. J Pathol 1998;185: 319-323.

[38] Corbel M, Caulet-Maugendre S, Germain N, Molet S, Lagente V, Boichot E. Inhibition of bleomycin-induced pulmonary fibrosis in mice by the matrix metalloproteinase inhibitor batimastat. J Pathol 2001;193: 538-545.

[39] Fukuda Y, Ishizaki M, Kudoh S, Kitaichi M Yamanaka N. Localization of matrix metalloproteinases-1, -2, and -9 and tissue inhibitor of metalloproteinase-2 in interstitial lung diseases. Lab Invest 1998;78: 687-698.

[40] Edwards ST, Cruz AC, Donnelly S, Dazin PF, Schulman ES, Jones KD, Wolters PJ, Hoopes C, Dolganov GM, Fang KC. c-Kit immunophenotyping and metalloproteinase expression profiles of mast cells in interstitial lung diseases. J Pathol 2005;206: 279-290.

[41] Balbin M, Fueyo A, Knauper V, Lopez JM, Alvarez J, Sanchez LM, Quesada V, Bordallo J, Murphy G, Lopez-Otin C. Identification and enzymatic characterization of

two diverging murine counterparts of human interstitial collagenase (MMP-1) expressed at sites of embryo implantation. J Biol Chem 2001;276: 10253-10262.

[42] Delaisse JM, Eeckhout Y, Neff L, Francois-Gillet C, Henriet P, Su Y, Vaes G, Baron R. (Pro)collagenase (matrix metalloproteinase-1) is present in rodent osteoclasts and in the underlying bone-resorbing compartment. J Cell Sci 1993;106: 1071-1082.

[43] Ouchi H, Fujita M, Ikegame S, Ye Q, Inoshima I, Harada E, Kuwano K, Nakanishi Y. The role of collagenases in experimental pulmonary fibrosis. Pulm. Pharmacol. Ther. 2008; 21: 401-408.

[44] Swiderski R, Dencoff J, Floerchinger C, Shapiro S, Hunninghake G. Differential expression of extracellular matrix remodeling genes in a murine model of bleomycin-induced pulmonary fibrosis. Am J Pathol 1998;152: 821-828.

[45] Fujita M, Ye Q, Ouchi H, Harada E, Inoshima I, Kuwano K, Nakanishi Y. Doxycycline attenuated pulmonary fibrosis induced by bleomycin in mice. Antimicrob Agents Chemother 2006;50: 739-743.

[46] Cook DN, Brass DM, Schwartz DA. A matrix for new ideas in pulmonary fibrosis. Am J Respir Cell Mol Biol 2002;27: 122-124.

[47] Lim S, Roche N, Oliver BG, Mattos W, Barnes PJ, Chung KF. Balance of matrix metallo-protease-9 and tissue inhibitor of metalloprotease-1 from alveolar macrophages in cigarette smokers. Regulation by interleukin-10. Am J Respir Crit Care Med 2000;162: 1355-1360.

[48] Dahlen B, Shute J, Howarth P. Immunohistochemical localisation of the matrix metalloproteinases MMP-3 and MMP-9 within the airways in asthma. Thorax 1999;54: 590-596.

[49] Vernooy JH, Dentener MA, van Suylen RJ, Buurman WA, Wouters EF. Intratracheal instillation of lipopolysaccharide in mice induces apoptosis in bronchial epithelial cells: no role for tumor necrosis factor-alpha and infiltrating neutrophils. Am J Respir Cell Mol Biol 2001;24: 569-576.

[50] Rowe SJ, Allen L, Ridger VC, Hellewell PG, Whyte MK. Caspase-1-deficient mice have delayed neutrophil apoptosis and a prolonged inflammatory response to lipopolysaccharide-induced acute lung injury. J Immunol 2002;169: 6401-6407.

[51] Fujita M, Harada E, Ikegame S, Ye Q, Ouchi H, Inoshima I, Kuwano K, Nakanishi Y. Doxycycline attenuated lung injury by its biological effect apart from its antimicrobial function. Pulm Pharmacol Ther 2007;20: 669-675.

[52] Wittels EH, Coalson JJ, Welch MH, Guenter CA. Pulmonary intravascular leukocyte sequestration. A potential mechanism of lung injury. Am Rev Respir Dis 1974;109: 502-509.

[53] Corteling R, Wyss D, Trifilieff A. In vivo models of lung neutrophil activation. Comparison of mice and hamsters. BMC Pharmacol 2002;2: 1.

[54] Hasday J, Dubin W, Fitzgerald T, Bascom R. Cigarettes are a rich source of bacterial endotoxin. Chest 1996;109: 63S-64S.

[55] Hasday JD, Bascom R, Costa JJ, Fitzgerald T, Dubin W. Bacterial endotoxin is an active component of cigarette smoke. Chest 1999;115: 829-835.

[56] Vernooy JH, Dentener MA, van Suylen RJ, Buurman WA, Wouters EF. Longterm intratracheal lipopolysaccharide exposure in mice results in chronic lung inflammation and persistent pathology. Am J Respir Cell Mol Biol 2002;26: 152-159.

[57] Brusselle GG, Bracke KR, Maes T, D'hulst AI, Moerloose KB, Joos GF, Pauwels RA. Murine models of COPD. Pulm Pharmacol Ther. 2006;19:155-65.

[58] Miyazaki Y, Araki K, Vesin C, Garcia I, Kapanci Y, Whitsett JA, Piguet PF, Vassalli P. Expression of a tumor necrosis factor-alpha transgene in murine lung causes lymphocytic and fibrosing alveolitis. A mouse model of progressive pulmonary fibrosis. J Clin Invest. 1995; 96: 250-259.

[59] Piguet PF, Collart MA, Grau GE, Kapanci Y, Vassalli P. Tumor necrosis factor/cachectin plays a key role in bleomycin-induced pneumopathy and fibrosis. J Exp Med 1989;170: 655-663.

[60] Fujita M, Shannon JM, Irvin CG, Fagan KA, Cool C, Augustin A, Mason RJ. Overexpression of tumor necrosis factor-a produces an increase in lung volumes and pulmonary hypertension. Am. J. Physiol. Lung Cell Mol. Physiol. 2001;280: L39-L49.

[61] Fujita M, Mason RJ, Cool C, Shannon JM, Hara N, Fagan KA. Pulmonary hypertension in TNF-alpha-overexpressing mice is associated with decreased VEGF gene expression. J Appl Physiol 2002;93: 2162-2170.

[62] Fujita M, Shannon JM, Morikawa O, Gauldie J, Hara N, Mason RJ. Overexpression of tumor necrosis factor-alpha diminishes pulmonary fibrosis induced by bleomycin or transforming growth factor-beta. Am J Respir Cell Mol Biol 2003;29: 669-676.

[63] Churg A, Wang RD, Tai H, Wang X, Xie C, Wright JL. Macrophage metalloelastase mediates acute cigarette smoke-induced inflammation via tumor necrosis factor-{alpha} release. Am J Respir Crit Care Med 2003;167: 1083-1089..

[64] Tang W, Geba GP, Zheng T, Ray P, Homer RJ,Kuhn C 3rd, Flavell RA, Elias JA. Targeted expression of IL-11 in the murine airway causes lymphocytic inflammation, bronchial remodeling, and airways obstruction. J Clin Invest 1996;98: 2845-2853.

[65] Kuhn C, 3rd, Homer RJ, Zhu Z, Ward N, Flavell RA, Geba GP, Elias JA. Airway hyperresponsiveness and airway obstruction in transgenic mice. Morphologic correlates in mice overexpressing interleukin (IL)-11 and IL-6 in the lung. Am J Respir Cell Mol Biol 2000;22: 289-295.

[66] Zhu Z, Homer RJ, Wang Z, Chen Q, Geba GP, Wang J, Zhang Y, Elias JA. Pulmonary expression of interleukin-13 causes inflammation, mucus hypersecretion, subepithelial fibrosis, physiologic abnormalities, and eotaxin production. J Clin Invest 1999;103: 779-788.

[67] Zheng T, Zhu Z, Wang Z, Homer RJ, Ma B, Riese RJ. Inducible targeting of IL-13 to the adult lung causes matrix metalloproteinase- and cathepsin-dependent emphysema. J Clin Invest 2000;106: 1081-1093.

[68] Wang Z, Zheng T, Zhu Z, Homer RJ, Riese RJ, Chapman HA Jr, Shapiro SD, Elias JA. Interferon gamma induction of pulmonary emphysema in the adult murine lung. J Exp Med 2000;192: 1587-1600.

[69] Wert SE, Yoshida M, LeVine AM, Ikegami M, Jones T, Ross GF, Fisher JH, Korfhagen TR, Whitsett JA. Increased metalloproteinase activity, oxidant production, and emphysema in surfactant protein D gene-inactivated mice. Proc Natl Acad Sci USA 2000;97: 5972–5977.

[70] Shibata Y, Zsengeller Z, Otake K, Palaniyar N, Trapnell BC. Alveolar macrophage deficiency in osteopetrotic mice deficient in macrophage colony-stimulating factor is spontaneously corrected with age and associated with matrix metalloproteinase expression and emphysema. Blood 2001;98: 2845–2852.

[71] Morris DG, Huang X, Kaminski N, Wang Y, Shapiro SD, Dolganov G, Glick A, Sheppard D. Loss of integrin alpha(v)beta6- mediated TGF-beta activation causes MMP12-dependent emphysema. Nature 2003;422: 169–173.

[72] Yoshida M, Korfhagen TR, Whitsett JA. Surfactant protein D regulates NF-kappa B and matrix metalloproteinase production in alveolar macrophages via oxidant-sensitive pathways. J Immunol 2001;166: 7514-7519.

[73] Shipley JM, Wesselschmidt RL, Kobayashi DK, Ley TJ, Shapiro SD. Metalloelastase is required for macrophage-mediated proteolysis and matrix invasion in mice. Proc Natl Acad Sci USA 1996; 93: 3942-3946.

[74] Hautamaki RD, Kobayashi DK, Senior RM, Shapiro SD. Requirement for macrophage elastase for cigarette smoke-induced emphysema in mice. Science 1997;277: 2002–2004.

[75] Shapiro SD, Goldstein NM, Houghton AM, Kobayashi DK, Kelley D, Belaaouaj A. Neutrophil elastase contributes to cigarette smoke-induced emphysema in mice. Am J Pathol 2003;163: 2329-2335.

[76] D'Armiento J, Dalal SS, Okada Y, Berg RA, Chada K. Collagenase expression in the lungs of transgenic mice causes pulmonary emphysema. Cell 1992;71: 955–961.

[77] Leco KJ, Waterhouse P, Sanchez OH, Gowing KL, Poole AR, Wakeham A, Mak TW, Khokha R. Spontaneous air space enlargement in the lungs of mice lacking tissue inhibitor of metalloproteinases-3 (TIMP-3). J Clin Invest 2001;108: 817–829.

[78] Lanone S, Zheng T, Zhu Z, Liu W, Lee CG, Ma B, Chen Q, Homer RJ, Wang J, Rabach LA, Rabach ME, Shipley JM, Shapiro SD, Senior RM, Elias JA. Overlapping and enzyme-specific contributions of matrix metalloproteinases-9 and -12 in IL-13-induced inflammation and remodeling. J Clin Invest 2002;110: 463–474.

[79] Balbín M, Fueyo A, Knäuper V, López JM, Alvarez J, Sánchez LM, Quesada V, Bordallo J, Murphy G, López-Otín C. Identification and enzymatic characterization of two diverging murine counterparts of human interstitial collagenase (MMP-1) expressed at sites of embryo implantation. J Biol Chem 2001;276: 10253–10262.

[80] Shapiro SD. Proteolysis in the lung. Eur Respir J Suppl 2003;44: 30s-32s.

[81] Imai K, Dalal SS, Chen ES, Downey R, Schulman LL, Ginsburg M, D'Armiento J. Human collagenase (matrix metalloproteinase-1) expression in the lungs of patients with emphysema. Am J Respir Crit Care Med 2001;163: 786-791

[82] Ohnishi K, Takagi M, Kurokawa Y, Satomi S, Konttinen YT. Matrix metalloproteinase-mediated extracellular matrix protein degradation in human pulmonary emphysema. Lab Invest 1998;78: 1077-1087.

[83] Betsuyaku T, Nishimura M, Takeyabu K, Tanino M, Venge P, Xu S, Kawakami Y. Neutrophil granule proteins in bronchoalveolar lavage fluid from subjects with subclin ical emphysema. Am J Respir Crit Care Med 1999;159: 1985-1991

[84] Finlay GA, Russell KJ, McMahon KJ, D'arcy EM, Masterson JB, FitzGerald MX, O'Connor CM. Elevated levels of matrix metalloproteinases in bronchoalveolar lavage fluid of emphysema tous patients. Thorax 1997;52: 502-506.

[85] Shapiro SD. Elastolytic metalloproteinases produced by human mononuclear phagocytes. Potential roles in destructive lung disease. Am J Respir Crit Care Med 1994;150: S160-164

[86] Segura-Valdez L, Pardo A, Gaxiola M, Uhal BD, Becerril C, Selman M. Upregulation of gelatin ases A and B, collagenases 1 and 2, and increased parenchymal cell death in COPD. Chest 2000;117: 684-694

[87] Han Z, Junxu, Zhong N. Expression of matrix metalloproteinases MMP-9 within the airways in asthma. Respir Med 2003;97: 563-567.

[88] Betsuyaku T, Tanino M, Nagai K, Nasuhara Y, Nishimura M, Senior RM. Extracellular matrix metalloproteinase inducer is increased in smokers' bronchoalveolar lavage fluid. Am J Respir Crit Care Med 2003;168: 222-227.

[89] Vignola AM, Riccobono L, Mirabella A, Profita M, Chanez P, Bellia V, Mautino G, D'accardi P, Bousquet J, Bonsignore G. Sputum metallo-proteinase-9/tissue inhibitor of metalloproteinase-1 ratio correlates with airflow obstruction in asthma and chronic bronchitis. Am J Respir Crit Care Med 1998;158: 1945-1950

[90] Choe KH, Taraseviciene-Stewart L, Scerbavicius R, Gera L, Tuder RM, Voelkel NF. Methylprednisolone causes matrix metalloproteinase-dependent emphysema in adult rats. Am. J. Respir. Crit. Care Med., 2003;167:1516-1521.

[91] Daheshia M. Therapeutic Inhibition of Matrix Metalloproteinases for the Treatment of Chronic Obstructive Pulmonary Disease (COPD) Curr Med Res Opin 2005;21: 587-594.

[92] Barnes PJ. New treatments for COPD. Nat Rev Drug Discov 2002;1: 437-446.

[93] Barnes PJ. New anti-inflammatory targets for chronic obstructive pulmonary disease. Nat Rev Drug Discov. 2013;12: 543-559.

[94] Churg A, Wang R, Wang X, Onnervik PO, Thim K, Wright JL. Effect of an MMP-9/ MMP-12 inhibitor on smoke-induced emphysema and airway remodelling in guinea pigs. Thorax 2007; 62: 706–713.

Chapter 4

Nature and Consequences of the Systemic Inflammatory Response Induced by Lung Inflammation

Kunihiko Hiraiwa and Stephan F. van Eeden

Additional information is available at the end of the chapter

http://dx.doi.org/10.5772/57392

1. Introduction

Lung inflammation is the basis for the majority of acute and chronic lung conditions. Acute lung injury (ALI) caused by either communicable (such as infection) or non-communicable (such as acid aspiration) diseases are characterized by a rapidly induced inflammatory response in the lung. There are numerous causes for ALI, as the lung is exposed to external factors either via the airways (infectious agents and environmental pollutants) or via the blood stream (sepsis, endotoxin, fat) and, when severe, can lead to acute respiratory distress syndrome (ARDS), a spectrum of lung diseases characterized by a severe inflammatory process in the lung parenchyma causing diffuse alveolar damage and respiratory failure [1, 2]. This acute inflammatory response in the lung is strongly associated with a systemic inflammatory response that may lead to multiple organ dysfunction and is associated with high mortality [3]. Similarly, chronic inflammatory lung conditions such as chronic obstructive pulmonary disease (COPD), asthma, bronchiectasis and interstitial lung diseases, especially those associated with collagen vascular disease, have in recent years also been shown to be accompanied by a systemic inflammatory response, albeit different in nature [4-14]. In addition, the systemic response induced by chronic lung inflammation is also associated with downstream adverse effects on different organ systems. This chapter will focus on defining the nature and features of this systemic response as a consequence of lung inflammation and will focus predominantly on chronic inflammatory lung conditions.

2. Lung conditions associated with a systemic inflammatory response

Numerous lung conditions, especially inflammatory lung conditions, are known to be associated with a systemic inflammatory response. Although the associations and consequences of the systemic response in acute lung injury and inflammation have been well established [1, 2, 15], the associations in chronic inflammatory lung conditions are less well known. This chapter will discuss the current knowledge surrounding inflammatory lung conditions and their associations with a systemic response.

2.1. Acute lung inflammation

The most recognized causes of acute lung inflammation are those induced either by infection or by direct or indirect ALI: for example, infections beginning in the lungs frequently transition into systemic events with hemodynamic effects (shock) and remote organ dysfunction such as acute kidney injury, which, when severe, may lead to death. Traditionally, the transition of infection from a localized event to one that is systemic in scope has been termed sepsis and is characterized by fever, tachycardia, tachypnea and a constellation of other signs and symptoms indicating that the pathogen and the humoral events that accompany the infectious process, are now systemically distributed. Furthermore, a number of publications suggest that clinical events such as severe tissue injury and ischemia-reperfusion injury may also activate the systemic response of the host in a similar manner to sepsis [16, 17]. The recognition of this common pathophysiologic phenotype of the sepsis syndrome led to the term "systemic inflammatory response syndrome" or SIRS, characterized by global activation of the inflammatory cascade, with an increase in circulating proinflammatory mediators leading to adverse downstream effects on numerous organ systems (so called multi-organ dysfunction). As mentioned, SIRS is an inflammatory response resulting from either local or systemic inflammatory events which may be initiated by either infectious or non-infectious insults [18, 19].

The local acute inflammatory response in the lung is complex and involves activation of the innate immune response via binding of microbial products or cell injury-associated endogenous molecules (danger-associated molecular patterns [DAMPs]) to pattern recognition receptors such as the toll-like receptors on the lung epithelium and alveolar macrophages [20]. Complex autocrine and paracrine inter-relationships exist between cytokines and other proinflammatory mediators such as endothelial adhesion molecules that both initiate and amplify the inflammatory response. This is augmented further by the margination and migration of polymorphonuclear neutrophils (PMNs) and other humoral responses, both dependent or independent of the cells, such as lipid mediators, proteases, oxidants, growth factors (such as transforming growth factors [TGFs]), nitric oxide and neuropeptides [21]. Increased permeability of microvascular barriers results in extravascular accumulation of protein-rich edema fluid in airspaces, a cardinal feature of acute inflammation and a central pathophysiologic mechanism in ALI/ARDS.

The local inflammatory insult in the lung may exceed the efficiency of the inflammatory response to effectively contain it, resulting in inflammatory elements of either bacterial cell products and toxins or cellular alarmins, pathogen-associated molecular patterns (PAMPs) and other inflammatory elements of the local response to gain systemic access in sufficient quantity to activate the systemic inflammatory response.

The magnitude of the insult is not the sole determining factor for host failure to contain the inflammatory response: in some instances, defects in the hosts' responses may contribute significantly. Host defects may be attributed to prior corticosteroid treatment, protein-calorie malnutrition or even genetic make-up, for example. The systemic response is characterized by activation of the coagulation cascade, complement proteins and the acute phase response.

Activation of cellular elements of blood such as platelets, granulocytes and mast cells cause degranulation and release of potent proinflammatory contents systemically, resulting in the systemic unleashing of otherwise beneficial local effects, leading to significant adverse effects on multiple extra-pulmonary organs.

2.2. Chronic lung inflammation

Since the 1970's and 1980's, the importance and consequences of the systemic response following acute lung inflammation have been recognized and well described, however, the systemic inflammatory response in chronic inflammatory lung conditions has only been recognized within the last ten years. The consequences and significance of this "lower grade" systemic response has only recently been more clearly defined. The chronic systemic inflammatory response in the lung is characterized by mobilization and activation of inflammatory cells into the circulation, the production of acute phase proteins and an increase in circulating inflammatory mediators. Of all the chronic inflammatory lung conditions, the systemic responses and consequences have been best characterized in COPD.

An integral component of the systemic inflammatory response is the stimulation of the hematopoietic system, specifically the bone marrow, which results in the release of leukocytes and platelets into the circulation. Large population-based studies have shown that the magnitude of the leukocytic response is a predictor of total mortality, independent of smoking [22-24].

Chronic cigarette smoking increases circulating leukocyte numbers [25, 26], including immature neutrophils, and results in high levels of myeloperoxidase and α_1-antitrypsin, the latter a natural inhibitor of serine proteases and responsible for alveolar wall damage [27, 28], suggesting that the systemic response feeds back to the lung and perpetuates the lung inflammatory response.

The acute phase response is an early and key part of the systemic component of the innate immune response and C-reactive protein (CRP) is a robust marker of this response. Subjects with severe airflow obstruction are more likely to have elevated CRP-levels and, in addition, high CRP levels have been related directly to severity of COPD and the associated systemic inflammation, independent of cigarette smoking and coronary artery disease [29-32].

Local anti-inflammatory therapy (inhaled corticosteroids) reduces circulating CRP whereas withdrawal of inhaled corticosteroids results in a significant increase in CRP levels [33], suggesting that lung inflammation drives the CRP levels in the blood of subjects with COPD. Moreover, CRP levels increase further during COPD exacerbations when lung inflammation flares up [33]. The increased circulating levels of CRP in COPD are associated with other mediators such as IL-6, which is the predominant cytokine regulator of CRP production by hepatocytes.

Lastly, subjects with COPD have higher levels of several circulating proinflammatory mediators such as tumor necrosis factor (TNF)-α and its receptors (TNFR-55 and -75), which are associated with leukocyte activation and the concomitant weight loss in these subjects [34-39]. Levels of the proinflammatory mediators IL-6 and IL-8 have also been shown to increase systemically during acute exacerbations of COPD [40, 41] suggesting that exacerbation of lung inflammation fuels the systemic response.

Chronic obstructive pulmonary disease is predominantly caused when the lung is exposed to noxious particulate matter and gases from cigarette smoke. Lung inflammation induced by inhalation of other air pollutants such as particulate matter or PM_{10}, nitric dioxide or ozone also causes a low grade inflammatory response in the lung. Experimental animal models exposed to ambient air pollutants [42, 43] and studies in humans [44, 45] have both shown that the inflammatory response in the lung induced by air pollutants is also associated with systemic inflammation, suggesting that the systemic response is not specific for cigarette smoke exposure (Figure 1).

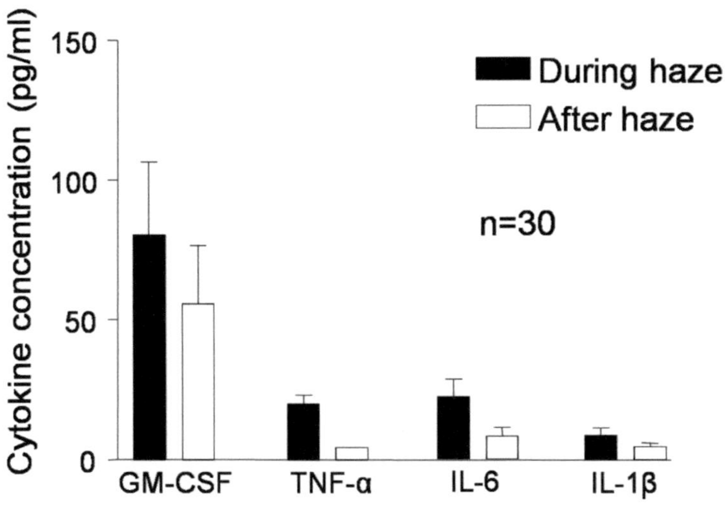

Figure 1. Cytokines in the blood of subject during the Southeast Asia forest fires of 1997. The black bars represent the concentrations of cytokines in the serum during the haze period and the white bars after the haze cleared. Cytokine levels were higher during haze compared with after haze. Values are mean ± SEM of all samples with values within the detection limit of the assay (n = 30 per group).

Similar to lung inflammation caused by inhalation exposure, the systemic response has also been well documented in other inflammatory lung conditions such as asthma [4-7], suppurative lung conditions such as bronchiectasis [8, 9], interstitial lung disease (ILD), in particular, ILD associated with collagen vascular diseases such as lupus erythematosus, rheumatoid arthritis and scleroderma [10-14]. As stated previously, these chronic inflammatory lung conditions are associated with increased levels of acute phase proteins such as CRP, stimulation of the bone marrow with altered circulating leukocyte and platelets and increased circulating proinflammatory mediators. Extensive studies have been undertaken to identify potential biomarkers capable of predicting disease severity and prognosis, implying that the systemic response to lung inflammation is an integral part of the disease and has important implications for disease pathogenesis and prognosis.

3. Lung cells contribute to the systemic inflammatory response induced by lung inflammation

The cells lining the airways are mainly epithelial cells but also include alveolar macrophages and both cell types are exposed to the external environment. They are the first responders in the lung when the lung is exposed to external factors such as cigarette smoke, air pollutants or infectious agents. These cells are critically important in the processing and neutralization of inhaled environmental contaminants which include airborne particulate matter (PM), cigarette smoke, bacteria and viruses, shown in Figure 2. Alveolar macrophages are one of the most potent producers of inflammatory mediators in the lung. It is known that human alveolar macrophages exposed to PM_{10} (EHC-93) [46] are able to phagocytose these particles *in vivo* [43] and *in vitro* [45] and produce, in a dose-dependent manner, an array of mediators such as IL-1β, IL-6 and TNF-α that are part of the innate immune response. To test the contribution of the mediators produced by alveolar macrophages to the systemic response, supernatants from alveolar macrophages, incubated *ex vivo* with urban PM, were instilled into the lungs of rabbits. The supernatants produced a systemic bone-marrow stimulation response similar to that produced by direct deposition of urban PM into the rabbit lung [42, 43]. Analysis of the supernatants showed that the proinflammatory mediators IL-1β and IL-6, the chemokine macrophage inflammatory protein (MIP)-1α and granulocyte macrophage colony-stimulating factor (GM-CSF) are elevated when macrophages are incubated with urban PM [45]. Studies showing a strong relationship between the quantity of particles phagocytosed by macrophages in lung tissue and the magnitude of the systemic response, after urban PM exposure (Figure 3), support the notion that the production of inflammatory mediators by alveolar macrophages is important and suggests that alveolar macrophages are significant contributors to the innate component of the systemic response following an inflammatory stimulus in the lung

Similar experiments using bronchial epithelial cells showed that, when exposed to urban PM, cells produce excess GM-CSF, IL-1β, IL-6, TNF-α, IL-8 and leukemia inhibitory factor (LIF) in a dose-dependent manner [47-49]. Some overlap was evident when comparing mediators produced by alveolar macrophages with those produced by bronchial epithelial cells after exposure to similar doses of urban PM, however, some distinct differences in the type and the magnitude of cytokine production was observed (Figure 4). The relative contributions of macrophages and epithelial cells in the production of mediators responsible for the systemic inflammatory response need to be determined. Alveolar macrophages are professional phagocytes and the magnitude of their cytokine production is significantly higher than bronchial epithelial cells, after the same level of exposure (Figure 4). These studies suggest that alveolar macrophages are key effector cells, responsible, at least, for generating the systemic inflammatory response associated with exposure to air pollution. However, although the macrophages are more potent producers of proinflammatory mediators expressed per cell basis, the airspace epithelial cells out-number the alveolar macrophages approximately ten

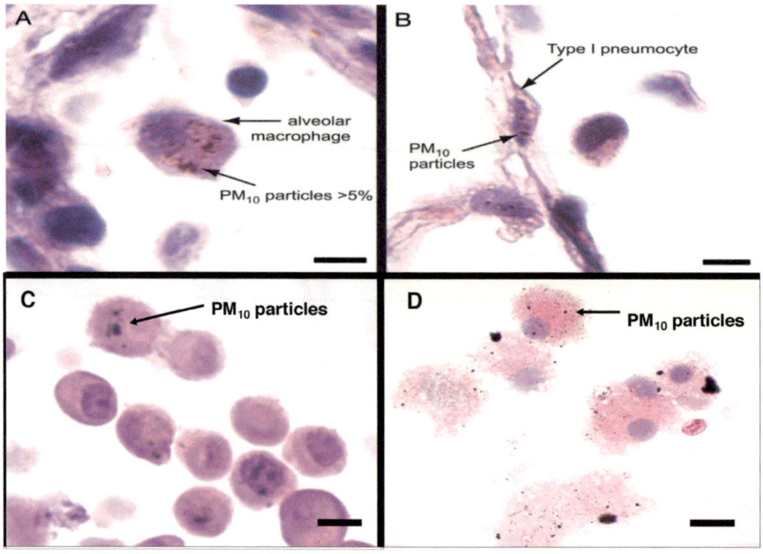

Figure 2. Photomicrographs of ambient particles phagocytosed by alveolar macrophages (A and D) and bronchial epithelial cells (B and C). **A and B:** Ambient particles (EHC-93] in alveolar macrophages (A) and both type I and type II epithelial cells (B) in rabbits exposed to 5 mg EHC-93 twice a week for 4 wks. **C:** Particles in primary cultures of human bronchial epithelial cells exposed to EHC-93 [100 µg/ml) for 24h. **D:** Particles in alveolar macrophages exposed to EHC-93 [100 µg/ml) for 24 h. The bar represents 10 µm [162].

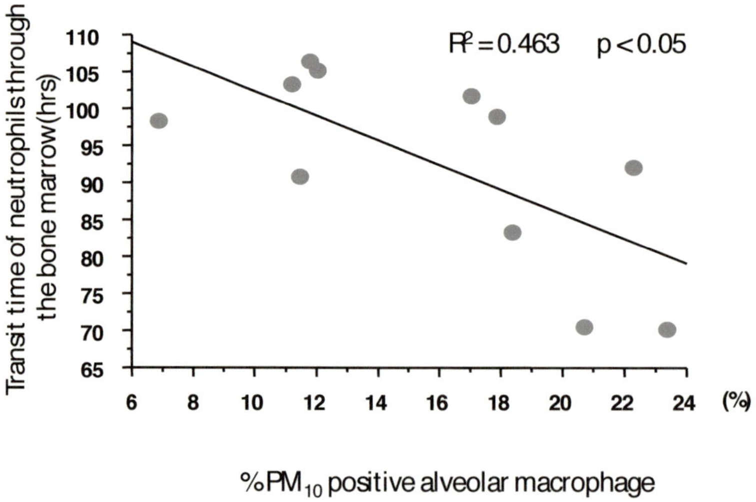

Figure 3. Relationship between the fraction of alveolar macrophages (AMs) that phagocytosed PM_{10} particles and the transit time of PMNs though the bone marrow. Rabbits were exposed to 5 mg PM_{10} (EHC-93) twice a week for 4 weeks, and AMs with particles in their cytoplasm were enumerated using quantitative histological methods. Dividing PMNs in the marrow were labeled with 5-bromo-2-deoxyuridine and the transit time of PMNs through the bone marrow was measured. Faster transit times of PMNs through the marrow were associated with an increased percentage of AMs with phagocytosed particles ($R^2 = 0.46$, $p < 0.05$) [162].

http://dx.doi.org/10.5772/57392

times. Furthermore, the interaction between macrophages and epithelial cells has a synergistic effect on the production and release of mediators involved in the systemic inflammatory response [50], therefore alveolar macrophages and airspace epithelial cells both play central roles in the activation of the innate immune response and the production of inflammatory mediators involved in the systemic response to lung inflammation.

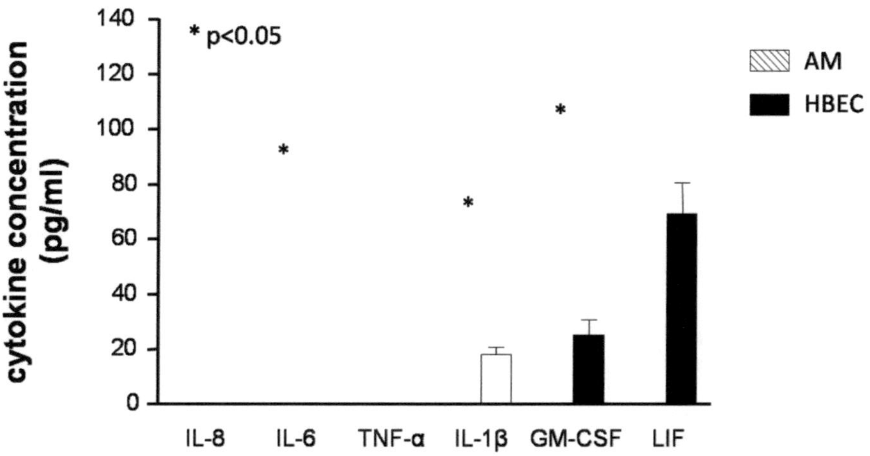

Figure 4. Cytokines produced by human AMs and bronchial epithelial cells (HBECs) when exposed to 100 μg/mL of PM_{10} (EHC-93] for 24 h. Differences between two groups were compared by Mann–Whitney U test. Alveolar macrophages produced significantly more IL-6, IL-1β and GM-CSF than bronchial epithelial cells when exposed to the same amount of PM_{10} [162].

The roles of other lung cells such as connective tissue cells (fibroblast, smooth muscle cells), immune cells (lymphocytes and dendritic cells) and vascular cells (endothelium) in the systemic response to lung inflammation are less clear. Several studies have documented increased levels of endothelial specific markers (soluble P, E and L-selectin, intercellular adhesion molecule [ICAM]-1, vascular cell adhesion molecule [VCAM]-1 and endothelin-1) present in the circulation during lung inflammation [51-53] but whether these mediators come directly from the lung or are released secondary to the initial circulating proinflammatory mediators such as IL-1β and TNF-α, is unclear. Mediators released from connective tissue cells and immune cells of the adaptive immune responses tend to be more localized in cellular niches with less of a systemic consequence.

4. Mediators of the systemic inflammatory response induced by lung inflammation

Lung inflammation has been associated with an array of different circulating cellular or non-cellular mediators that may differ significantly depending on the type and the character of the inflammatory response in the lung.

4.1. Cellular components of the systemic response to lung inflammation

Increased circulating leukocyte counts, specifically granulocyte counts, have been used for decades as biomarkers of local inflammatory or infectious processes, including lung inflammation. Large population-based studies showing leukocytosis as a predictor of total mortality, independent of other risk factors such as cigarette smoking, underline the importance of increases in circulating leukocytes [23, 54, 55]. Therefore, an integral component of the systemic response to lung inflammation is the stimulation of the hematopoietic system, specifically the bone marrow, which results in an increase in circulating leukocytes. In humans, leukocyte increases caused by bone marrow stimulation can be identified and quantified by an increase in circulating immature granulocytes (band cells and metamyelocytes) [42], in contrast to increases in leukocyte counts induced by exercise or other cathecholamine stress that results largely in demargination of existing intravascular leukocytes [56]. When associated with lung inflammation, an increase in circulating band cells signifies that signals from the lung have activated and stimulated the bone marrow to release immature leukocytes. In humans both acute lung inflammation such as pneumonia [57] and chronic lung inflammation such as exposure to cigarette smoke or other air pollutants [44] have been shown to increase circulating band cells counts, implicating a systemic response that stimulates the bone marrow. In contrast, two separate studies of healthy subjects residing in regions with low particulate air pollution (such as the South Pole) for prolonged periods, showed that the circulating white blood cell (WBC) count fell below the normal range shortly after the subjects entered this pristine environment, remained low for the entire period that they were in this environment, and then returned to normal levels when they returned to the either the US [58] or Japan [59]. The Japanese study also showed that the fall in circulating leukocytes was associated with a fall in the number of circulating band cells, indicating a reduction in bone marrow output [59]. These studies suggest that the reductions in circulating WBC and band cell counts are the result of a reduction in bone marrow stimulation initiated by signals generated in the lung. To more accurately quantify the bone marrow response to lung inflammation, one group has developed a method to label precursor cells in the marrow with the thymidine analogue 5'bromo-2-deoxyuridine (BrdU) [60-62], allowing accurate identification of newly released leukocytes from the bone marrow and simplifying functional studies. Using this method they demonstrated that acute lung inflammation caused by a focal infection [61], as well as chronic lung inflammation induced by either cigarette smoke or urban air pollutants [27, 42, 63, 64], stimulate the bone marrow and accelerates the transit times of granulocytes and monocytes through the marrow, releasing them into the circulating pool of leukocytes. The ability to follow these labeled cells in the circulation allowed study of cell behavior and functional capability whereby this group was able to show preferential sequestration of younger PMNs in the gravity independent lung regions of animals exposed to cigarette smoke [63] and less efficient migration into inflammatory sites, compared to more mature cells [65, 66]. *In vitro* studies support these findings, showing that younger PMNs released from the bone marrow are less deformable and less chemotactic than mature PMNs already in the circulation [67].

Collectively, these studies have established that the circulating blood contains granulocytes such as neutrophils of varying ages and functional capabilities and that lung inflammation-

http://dx.doi.org/10.5772/57392

induced bone marrow stimulation increases the population of younger PMN with a greater potential to damage tissue (Figure 5). This knowledge may be relevant to the pathogenesis of acute lung inflammation-induced adverse organ dysfunction in conditions such as sepsis, or the systemic adverse effects associated with chronic inflammatory lung conditions such as COPD. The immature leukocytes also tend to preferentially sequester in lung capillaries [65, 67] where they may further damage the lung and fuel lung inflammation, causing a vicious cycle of lung inflammation leading to systemic inflammation that feeds back, resulting in further lung inflammation (Figure 5). It is possible that the bone marrow stimulation associated with both acute and chronic inflammatory lung conditions contributes to the development of acute lung injury such as in ARDS as well as chronic lung injury promoting centrilobular emphysema in susceptible subjects.

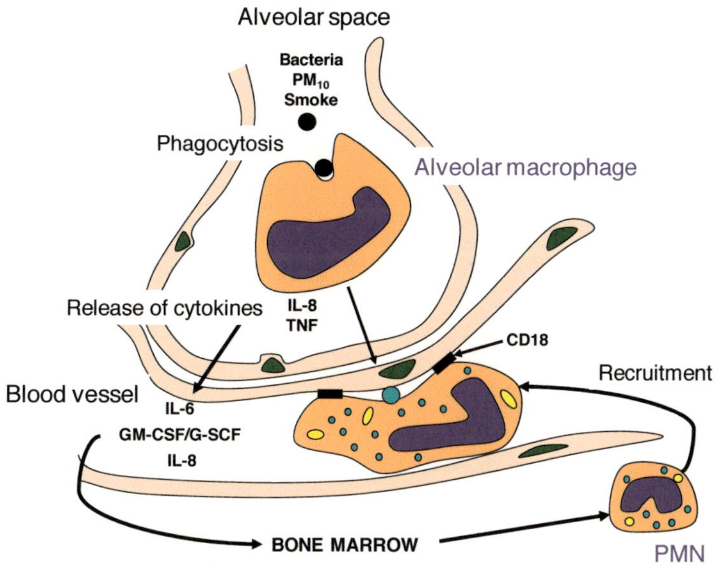

Figure 5. Lung injury induced by immature PMNs. Alveolar macrophages and epithelial cells phagocytose bacteria, particulate matter or cigarette smoke and induce cytokine production. These cytokines spill over into the circulation and stimulate the bone marrow to recruit leukocytes. The newly recruited immature PMNs tend to preferentially sequester in lung capillaries where they may be activated and degranulate, further damaging the lung. Lung damage leads to excess cytokine production which further fuels the systemic inflammation.

4.2. Non-cellular components of systemic response to lung inflammation

Common to nearly all inflammatory lung conditions are the production and release of mediators of the innate immune response. These circulating mediators, specifically the "acute response" cytokines IL-1β, IL-6 and TNF-α, activate the acute-phase response [68], by stimulating the liver to produce acute phase proteins, such as fibrinogen, that increases blood coagulability, which is a major risk factor for acute cardiovascular events in susceptible individuals [69]. Another acute-phase protein, CRP, is strongly associated with inflammation in general but, in epidemiological studies, has also been correlated with the extent of atherosclerosis and heart disease [29, 70]. C-reactive protein has become the hallmark biomarker indicative of the extent and severity of cardiovascular disease [71-73] as well as many other systemic inflammatory conditions, for example auto-immune collagen vascular diseases such as rheumatoid arthritis and lupus erythematosus. The acute response is a specific, well-orchestrated sequence of events, characterized by an early release of the "alarm" cytokines IL-1β and TNF-α, followed by a second wave of cytokines (IL-8, IL-6, monocyte chemotactic protein [MCP]-1 and MIP-1α) and growth factors such as GM-CSF and G-CSF. The second wave of cytokines produced in the lung is of particular importance in inducing the systemic inflammatory response. Granulocyte macrophage colony-stimulating factor is a hematopoietic growth factor that stimulates granulocyte and monocyte differentiation and release from the bone marrow, activates circulating leukocytes such as neutrophils and prolongs leukocyte survival in the circulation and tissues [74]. In addition, GM-CSF has also recently been identified as an important granulocyte deganulation factor that may enhance tissue damage induced by granulocytes [75]. One of the "acute response" cytokines that induces cytokine production by many cells is IL-1β, which is known to stimulate hematopoiesis, activate endothelial cells, induce the acute-phase response and is pyrogenic [76]. Similarly, IL-6 stimulates hepatocytes to produce acute phase proteins, including CRP, fibrinogen and antiproteases [77], stimulates hematopoiesis, specifically the production of platelets and has a broad stimulating effect on B- and T-cells. In addition, IL-6 activates the bone marrow, accelerates the transit time of granulocytes through the bone marrow promotes their release into the circulation and increases their sequestration in microvascular beds [78]. All the acute-phase response cytokines are proinflammatory in nature and suppress the production of anti-inflammatory cytokines such as IL-10, in fact, low circulating levels of this cytokine have been associated with a poor outcome in sepsis [79, 80]. Collectively, the acute response cytokines have the ability to elicit a systemic inflammatory response in response to lung inflammation that is characterized by an increase in circulating leukocytes, platelets and pro-inflammatory and prothrombotic mediators. In addition, cytokines also have the ability to activate circulating leukocytes and platelets, as well as vascular endothelium, to promote leukocyte–endothelial adhesion and migration into tissues.

Part of the lung injury or initial stress insult in the lung is the formation and release of microparticles (MP), which are small vesicles (0.1–1 mm in diameter) containing cell membrane, that are released by a variety of cells types following either activation or an insult such as oxidative stress [81]. Platelets, endothelial cells, leukocytes, erythrocytes and tumor cells are cell types prone to MP shedding. Microparticles are composed of cell membranes, with receptors, enclosing cytosolic components, including enzymes, transcription factors, mRNA and microRNA, all derived from the parent cell. Microparticles contain signaling elements that may activate receptors on target cells and may also bind to target cells and transfer part of their contents [82]. Moreover, because MPs circulate, they not only act on their local environment but also on sites far from their origin, thereby serving as a cell-to-cell communication network. Microparticles are known to affect inflammation, coagulation, endothelial function, cell survival, and intercellular communication [81].

Moreover, they have been documented at sites of inflammation [83, 84] and increased numbers of circulating MPs have been reported in systemic diseases such as autoimmune collagen vascular disorders, atherosclerosis, hypercoagulability states, disseminating malignancies and infection, among others [85, 86]. Circulating endothelial MPs are associated with activated, damaged or stressed endothelial cells and are biomarkers of vascular injury. Microparticles may also remotely induce endothelial dysfunction by altering the intracellular production of vasorelaxing molecules such as nitric oxide and contributing to the recruitment of leukocytes at the remote site [81, 87, 88]. Recently, MPs have been shown to increase during inflammatory lung conditions such as COPD [89] and increase further during acute COPD exacerbations [90]. Furthermore, subjects with autoimmune collagen vascular disorders with lung involvement have increased levels of circulating endothelial MPs [91], suggesting that MPs are not just useful biomarkers of lung inflammation, but may play a critically important role in the pathogenesis of the downstream adverse effects that lung inflammation appears to have on distant organs.

5. Mechanisms of lung inflammation-induced systemic inflammation

Several mechanisms have been postulated to explain the association of lung inflammation with the systemic inflammatory response (Figure 6). The hypothesis with the most supporting experimental evidence postulates that inflammatory mediators generated in lung tissue translocate into the circulation. As the lung receives substantial cardiac output, it is reasonable to suppose that small molecules may translocate from lung tissue to the blood stream, following a natural gradient, a process that may be augmented by increases in capillary permeability which often accompanies the lung inflammatory process. It has been suggested that a gradient of the acute proinflammatory mediator, elastase, and its natural inhibitor, α1-anti-trypsin, forms across the lung during acute neutrophilic lung inflammation [92] and "spills over" into the systemic circulation. Recent studies from another group has confirmed these findings in experimental models of acute (lipopolysaccharides [LPS]-induced) and chronic (air pollution-induced) lung inflammation [93, 94], supporting the hypothesis that the lung *per se* contribute directly to the systemic inflammatory response associated with lung inflammation.

There is also some evidence indicating that triggers of lung inflammation, such as ultrafine particulate matter, LPS and other bacterial toxins, translocate from the airspaces to the bloodstream [84, 95-97], either directly contributing to the systemic response or stimulating circulating immune cells such as monocytes to produce proinflammatory mediators that contribute to the systemic response. Collectively, there is ample evidence that small molecules or particles have the ability to directly translocate from the lung into the blood stream, generating a systemic inflammatory response. This is a particularly important mechanism if vascular permeability is compromised during the lung inflammatory response because it will accelerate the systemic inflammatory response caused by lung inflammation.

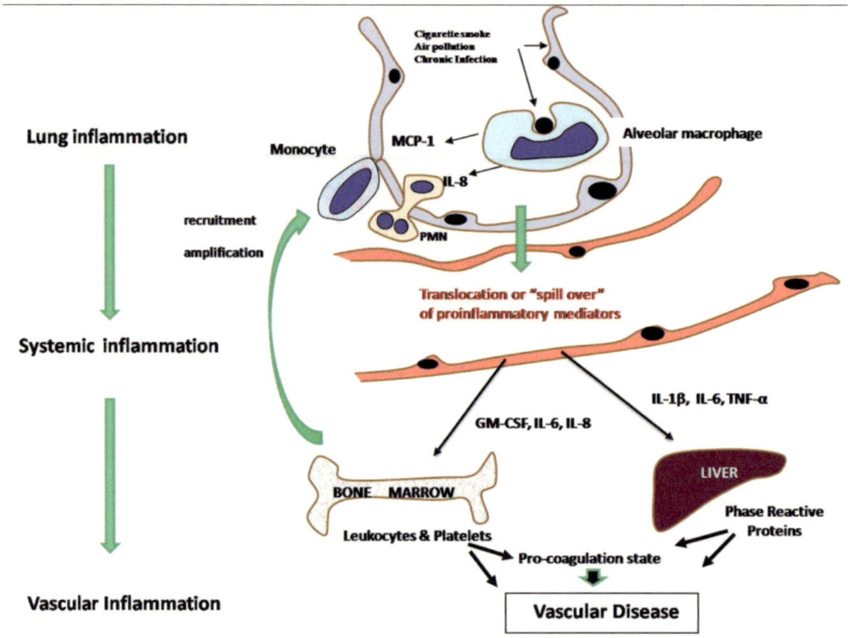

Figure 6. Impact of pulmonary inflammation on distant organ systems. Inflammatory mediators generated in the lung "spill over" into the circulation, activating the liver to release acute-phase proteins and the bone marrow to release leukocytes and platelets. Together, these circulating effector proteins and cells promote vascular disease and may precipitate acute vascular events. Systemic inflammation also enhances lung inflammation by promoting the recruitment of immune cells into lung tissues.

5.1. Feedback of downstream effects of the systemic response to acute lung inflammation

Bacterial or viral lung infections are common causes of acute lung inflammation that lead to ALI/ARDS [1]. During the past decade, novel and highly virulent respiratory viruses such as the Severe Acute Respiratory Syndrome Coronavirus (SARS CoV) and highly pathogenic strains of influenza viruses have emerged as important causes of excessive lung damage in infected humans. Acute lung injury and associated inflammation frequently have systemic manifestations, coined the "systemic inflammatory response syndrome (SIRS)". Many patients with refractory ALI/ARDS succumb to multiple organ failure (MOF) rather than respiratory failure, underlining the importance of the systemic response to lung injury. Many studies have been undertaken to investigate the cellular or molecular mechanisms of acute lung injury-induced systemic manifestations [1, 2, 15]. The deterioration from ALI/ARDS to MOF involves many steps, including the activation of multiple inflammatory pathways, increased expression of chemoattractants which results in endothelial changes and the release of proinflammatory cytokines such as IL-1β, IL-6 and TNF-α, margination and migration of neutrophils as well as systemic activation of monocytes, all contributing to diffuse microvascular injury which is thought to lead to multi-organ injury and eventual failure [98]. Currently it is thought that the pivotal injury occurs to the vascular endothelium, leading to increased vascular permeability, which is then followed by translocation of inflammatory mediators and activated leukocytes into organ tissue resulting in organ inflammation and, finally, dysfunction. Organs particular vulnerable to microvascular dysfunction are the kidney, liver, brain and the gastrointestinal system. Containing the lung inflammatory response is critically important in order to inhibit progression to a systemic inflammatory response fueled by the vicious cycle of increased cytokine production and cellular damage, underlining the importance of lung inflammation as the primary "driver" for the downstream multiple organ dysfunction.

5.2. Chronic lung inflammation and vascular dysfunction

Circulating cytokines produced in the lung activate the vascular endothelium and this activation is associated with increased expression of several adhesion proteins such as ICAM-1, VCAM-1 and E-selectin. Both soluble ICAM-1 and VCAM-1 are upregulated in circulating blood during chronic inflammation and are correlated with increased disease in coronary and carotid arteries in humans. Support of these observations comes from animal models that have shown instillation of atmospheric particles into the lungs of rabbits [99] and mice [100] results in development of atherosclerosis, followed by rapid progression of the atherosclerotic process over the surface of the aorta with concomitant destabilization of existing atherosclerotic plaques (Figure 7). Furthermore, particulate deposition in murine lungs is associated with upregulation of both ICAM-1 and VCAM-1 on the endothelium overlying the atherosclerotic plaques [101]. In addition, the number of particle-phagocytosing alveolar macrophages shows a strong positive association with the extent of atherosclerosis (Figure 8), as well as with markers of systemic inflammation such as CRP [102]. These studies demonstrate that lung inflammation stimulates alveolar macrophages, increases circulating markers of inflammation, increases endothelial activation and dysfunction and suggests a cause and effect relationship between lung inflammation and the development and progression of vascular diseases such as atherosclerosis.

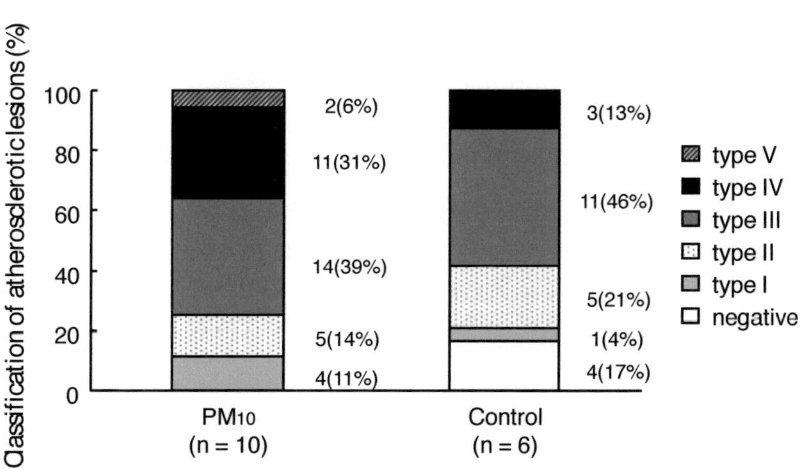

Figure 7. The severity of atherosclerotic lesions in the aorta. Results shown in rabbits exposed to PM_{10} for four weeks (n = 10) or saline (controls; n = 6). The classification is based on the guidelines of the American Heart Association (AHA) [163, 164]. PM_{10} exposure was associated with progression to more advanced phenotypes of atherosclerosis compared with the control group.

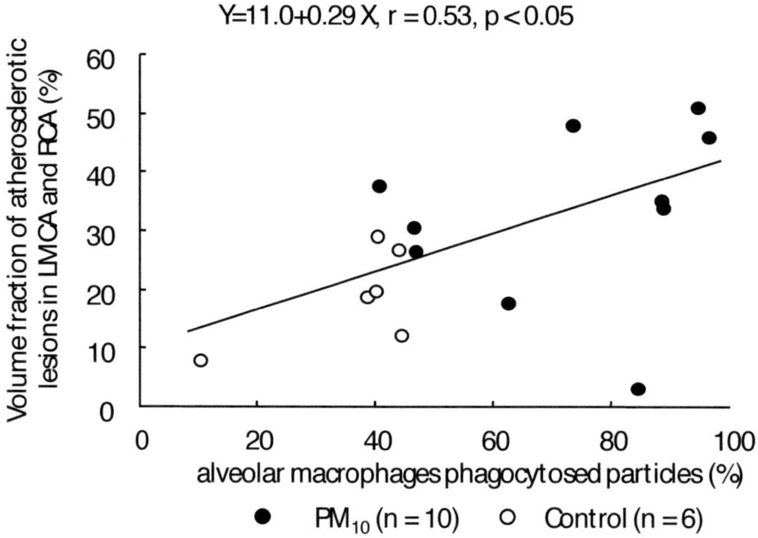

Figure 8. The correlation between the percentage of alveolar macrophages that phagocytosed particles in the lung and the vol/vol (volume fraction) of atherosclerotic lesions in the left main coronary artery (LMCA) and right coronary artery (RCA). Results shown in rabbits exposed to PM_{10} for four weeks (solid circles; n = 10) or saline (controls; open circles; n = 6). The volume fraction (vol/vol) of atherosclerosis was determined by point counting the sections. The correlation between variables were examined by the Spearman rank correlation test ($r = 0.53$, $p < 0.05$) [99].

5.3. Systemic inflammation in COPD

Numerous studies have established that COPD is associated with a low-grade systemic inflammatory response, which has been implicated in the pathogenesis of the majority of the systemic effects associated with COPD, including muscle weakness, weight loss, cardiovascular disease, depression, diabetes and osteoporosis [103]. Patients with stable COPD have increased numbers of circulating leukocytes, increased levels of acute phase response proteins (CRP and fibrinogen) and increased cytokine levels (IL-6 and TNF-α) [104] that increase further with acute exacerbations [105, 106].

Chronic obstructive pulmonary disease is a chronic inflammatory condition of the airways and lung parenchyma caused predominantly by the inhalation of toxic particles and noxious gasses, with cigarette smoking contributing to the bulk of the disease burden. There is a strong association between cardiovascular disease and COPD morbidity and mortality. Cardiovascular events are the predominant reason for hospitalizations (morbidity) and a leading cause of mortality in subjects with mild and moderate COPD [107]. Furthermore, epidemiological studies have shown that compromised lung function (FEV1) in subjects with COPD is associated with cardiovascular morbidity and mortality, even after controlling for smoking history [107], suggesting that the inflammatory response in the lung which causes the reduced lung function also impacts the vasculature. The mechanisms of COPD-induced cardiovascular disease are still unclear, however, animals models of cigarette exposure or exposure to ambient particulate matter suggest that the systemic response induced by these inhalation stimuli causes vascular dysfunction that may promote the development and progression of atherosclerotic vascular disease [99-102]. Activation of coronary vasculature by the systemic response to COPD lung inflammation also impacts other vascular beds such as the cerebral vascular bed. Circulating inflammatory mediators such as IL-1β, IL-6, TNF-α, α1-antichymotrypsin and TNFR1 are associated with cognitive decline, either through a direct neurotoxic effect or through cerebral atherosclerosis effects [108, 109]. Figure 9 highlights potential pathways of blood vessel activation due to systemic inflammation in COPD that results in endothelial dysfunction and destabilization of atherosclerotic plaques, possibly leading to vascular events such as acute coronary syndrome and stroke.

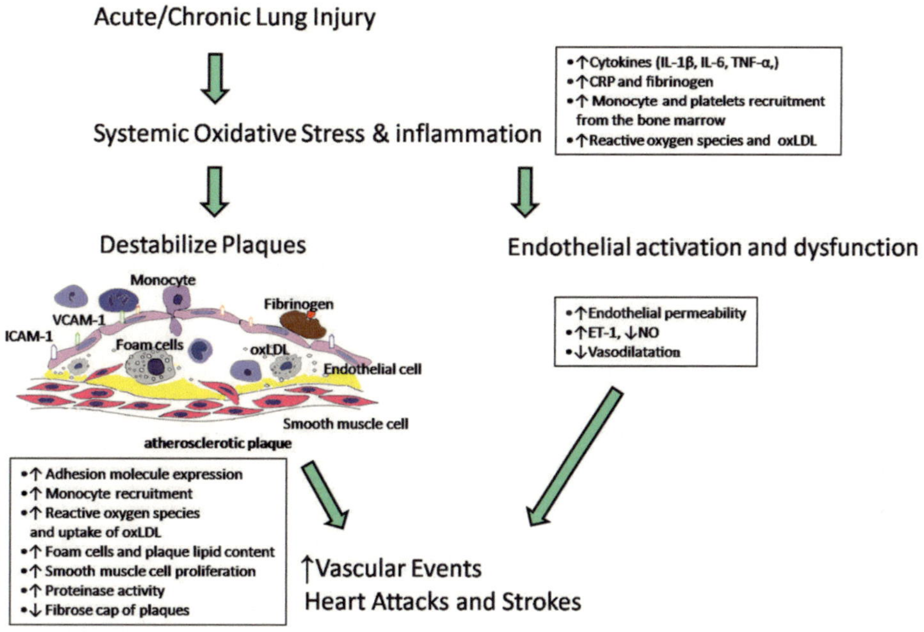

Figure 9. Impact of lung injury on blood vessels. Circulating mediators such as IL-6 induce the release of CRP and fibrinogen from the liver. In addition, IL-6 and GM-CSF stimulate the bone marrow to release leukocytes and platelets, while TNF-α and IL-1β activate vascular endothelial cells and upregulate endothelial ICAM-1 and VCAM-1, thereby promoting the recruitment of monocytes into blood vessel walls. Activation of endothelial cells also increases endothelial permeability, promotes uptake of oxidized low-density lipoproteins (oxLDL) into vessel walls, promotes the release of endothelin-1 (ET-1) and decreases availability of nitric oxide (NO). Together, these changes in blood vessel walls lead to endothelial dysfunction and promote vulnerability of atherosclerotic plaques to rupture, possibly leading to acute cardiac events or strokes.

Cachexia and muscle wasting are hallmarks of COPD, especially in subjects with severe disease and, currently, the mechanisms underlying these downstream effects of COPD are a topic of active investigation. In COPD subjects, skeletal muscle shows increased apoptosis, increased oxidative stress and increased inflammatory cell infiltration [110, 111], suggesting that inflammatory processes play a role in the physiologic changes seen in skeletal muscles of COPD subjects. Furthermore, the underlying inflammatory and oxidative processes in the lungs, in addition to the downstream proinflammatory systemic responses, shifts the hormonal balance towards catabolism, reducing testosterone levels and increasing catecholamine synthesis, especially in the severe stages of the disease (FEV1<30%) [112]. It is reasonable to postulate that the systemic inflammatory response associated with COPD lung inflammation contributes to the skeletal muscle inflammation and concomitant muscle wasting seen in COPD.

Both diabetes mellitus type2 and osteoporosis are associated with COPD, especially in subjects with greater disease severity [113-115]. The mechanisms underlying the former two diseases are complex but a postulated mechanisms linking them with COPD is the presence of elevated circulating levels of proinflammatory mediators such as IL-1β, IL-6 and TNF-α. Therefore it seems reasonable to postulate that the systemic response in COPD may either aggravate or enhance the development of osteoporosis and diabetes, to a certain extent.

5.4. Systemic inflammation in other inflammatory lung conditions

Asthma is predominantly an inflammatory condition of the airways, however a systemic inflammatory response has also been well documented, evidenced by an increase in circulating proinflammatory cytokines such as IL-6 and TNF-α that stimulate hepatic production of acute-phase proteins such as CRP, as well as an increase in immune cells such as neutrophils and eosinophils [4, 116]. Circulating TNF-α and IL-6 levels are further elevated during asthma exacerbation [117, 118]. Downstream consequences of this systemic response are less well studied and are insufficiently understood, therefore require further investigation. Similarly, interstitial lung disease and fibrosis are a large group of inflammatory lung conditions that include chronic hypersensitivity pneumonitis, sarcoidosis, drug-induced lung disease, lung disease associated with collagen vascular disease, idiopathic pulmonary fibrosis (IPF) and more. Many of these lung conditions are associated with increased circulating levels of pro-inflammatory mediators such as IL-1β, IL-6, TNF-α, TGF-β and platelet-derived growth factor (PDGF) [119, 120]. In conditions that exclusively involve the lung such as hypersensitivity pneumonitis and IPF, translocation of these mediators from the lung into the circulation may be responsible for the measured systemic response, however the effect of these mediators on other organ systems are unclear and require further study.

5.5. Effect of the systemic inflammatory response on lung inflammation

It is well known that non-pulmonary disorders (for example sepsis, trauma, massive transfusion, drug overdose, pancreatitis) cause lung injury and inflammation. "Crosstalk" between lungs and distal organs is an emerging, interesting and clinically relevant field [121, 122]. A complex network of cytokines, as well as proinflammatory chemokines such as CXCL1, from distant organs can initiate and amplify the lung injury [123, 124]. Many of the mediators involved in the systemic response have the ability to both damage lungs directly and stimulate the bone marrow to release leukocytes into the circulation. In addition, leukocytes that may have been sequestered in the lung could be released, potentially causing additional lung injury [125, 126]. These newly released leukocytes, specifically granulocytes such as neutrophils, have been shown to be preferentially sequestered in the pulmonary capillary bed where, if activated, they may contribute to further lung injury and damage [65, 66].

Patients afflicted with lung injury more commonly than not encounter more than 'one-hit' modulating the immunological response to injury by increasing duration and amplitude of the inflammatory response [127]. In animal models, the traditional "single-hit" model is no longer considered a good approximation of human ALI/ARDS, whereas a "two-hit" model has been shown to increase the inflammatory response in the lung [127-130]. This "priming" phenomenon may be pivotal in subjects with chronic lung inflammation, such as COPD, where the systemic inflammatory response induced by the chronic lung inflammation may feed-back, aggravating the lung inflammatory response. This vicious cycle of inflammation promoting further inflammation may be the reason why subjects with COPD still have active lung inflammation many years after they have stopped smoking [131]. This phenomenon is also seen in patients with asthma, where, even years after cessation of exposure, patients with Western red cedar-initiated asthma have persistent airflow obstruction [132]. In this study, higher impairment was associated with serum IFN-γ (Figure 10), which supports the hypothesis of a vicious cycle of inflammation with crosstalk between the lung and systemic inflammatory responses.

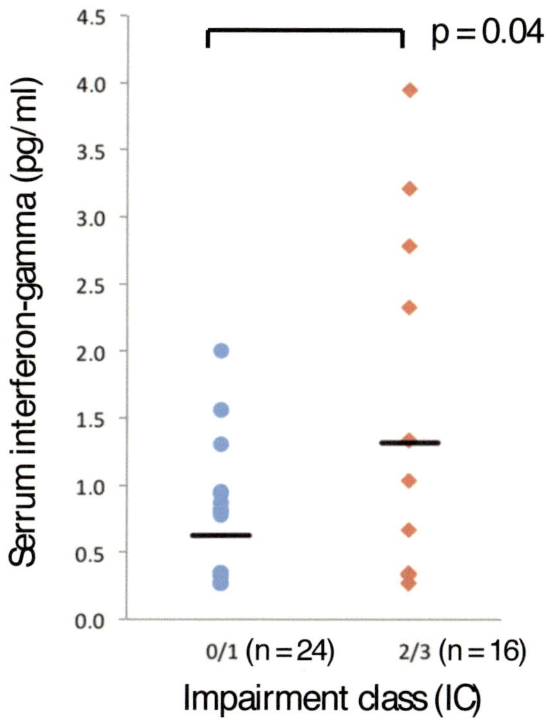

Figure 10. Serum interferon-gamma, stratified by higher (2/3) versus lower (0/1) respiratory impairment (IC = impairment class). The blood samples were collected from 40 non-smoking male at a mean interval of 25 years from cedar asthma diagnosis and 17 years from last cedar exposure. The respiratory impairment class was defined by ATS guidelines [165]. Asthma-related respiratory impairment was associated with higher interferon-gamma levels in serum (average 1.32 pg/ml for IC2/3 versus average 0.62 pg/ml for IC0/1; p = 0.04) [132].

6. Therapeutic alterations of lung inflammation-induced systemic responses

The mediators of systemic responses to lung inflammation are clinically useful tools with which to grade the severity of lung inflammation or to use as biomarkers for following the progression of the disease. Neutralization of these mediators using effector molecules termed "immunoresolvents" may prove useful in attenuating the downstream consequences of the systemic inflammatory response. Potential advantages of immunoresolvents lie in the possibilities of both attenuating leukocyte activation and decreasing recruitment into tissues, thereby reducing organ damage. However, in a study with more than 10,000 patients with sepsis, anti-inflammatory agents designed to inhibit specific host mediators, for example anti-TNF antibodies and IL-1 receptor antagonists, failed to show benefit, despite promising preclinical testing [133]. Similarly, another multicenter, randomized, double-blind study in patients with moderate to severe COPD showed that infliximab (anti-TNF-α monoclonal antibody) had no therapeutic benefit in reducing acute exacerbation of COPD [134]. Although many proinflammatory neutralizing therapies have the potential to be useful, they also evoke some unwanted effects, for example, TNF-specific antibody therapy reduces TNF-α concentrations but is also associated with increased susceptibility to infections and malignancies [134]. Clearly, immunosuppression is a critical drawback to some treatments and new therapeutics targeting resolution of inflammation would be required to circumvent this side effect.

The anti-inflammatory cytokine IL-10 balances the proinflammatory response and serves to limit and terminate the cascade of proinflammatory cytokines. Research shows that treatment with IL-10 reduces neutrophil and leukocyte recruitment and decreases proinflammatory cytokine-production in lung inflammation [135-138], underlining the importance of balancing the acute inflammatory response and suggesting that treatment using a combination of different therapeutic agents to alter outcome in the systemic inflammatory milieu may be more successful.

Recently several classes of pro-resolving mediators have been identified, including resolvins, protectins and maresins [139]. These specialized lipid mediators are derived via enzymatic processing from dietary omega-3 polyunsaturated fatty acids and have anti-inflammatory activity in lung inflammation [140, 141].

Originally designed to lower cholesterol, the 3-hydroxy-3-methylglutaryl coenzyme A (HMG-CoA) reductase class of drugs, also called "statins", are recognized as anti-inflammatory agents [142]. Experimental observations suggest that these agents have pleiotropic anti-inflammatory properties *in vitro* including the inhibition of isoprenoid synthesis, which leads to the inhibition of small proinflammatory signaling GTPases such as Rho, Rac and Cdc42 [143, 144]. Animal studies have demonstrated that statins attenuate lung injury in ischemia-reperfusion, peritonitis and aerosolized LPS models [145-147]. In addition, statins downregulate the PM_{10}-induced overactive bone marrow by attenuating systemic inflammatory responses such as the recruitment and activation of alveolar macrophages and polymorphonuclear leukocytes, as well as reducing local proinflammatory cytokine production and promoting the clearance of PM_{10} particles from lung tissues to regional lymph nodes [148, 149].

Several observational studies suggest that statins may represent a useful therapeutic adjunctive modality for ALI/ARDS: a benefit of prior statin use was found in patients with pneumonia [150-152]. Similarly, other studies showed a reduction in the frequency of COPD exacerbations, hospitalization, and mortality after statin therapy, which may be a result of a direct effect on lung inflammation, an impact on the systemic consequences of COPD, or both [153-161]. These studies indicate that statins are effective in decreasing lung and systemic inflammation in humans *in vivo*.

7. Conclusion

A systemic response is a hallmark of both acute and chronic lung inflammatory conditions. The nature and magnitude of this systemic response differs depending on the nature and magnitude of the inflammatory response in the lung. Mediators generated in the lung as part of the lung inflammatory response, translocate to the systemic circulation, contributing to the systemic response. This systemic response has significant downstream adverse consequences on distant organs suggesting it is as an important therapeutic target. Therapeutic tools to modify and alter the systemic response induced by lung conditions, are still lacking and need further study.

Acknowledgements

The authors acknowledge Dr. Katherine Thain for writing assistance.

Author details

Kunihiko Hiraiwa and Stephan F. van Eeden*

*Address all correspondence to: stephan.vaneeden@hli.ubc.ca

Department of Medicine, UBC James Hogg Research Centre, St. Paul's Hospital, University of British Columbia, Vancouver, Canada

References

[1] Ware LB, Matthay MA. The acute respiratory distress syndrome. N Engl J Med. 2000 May 4;342(18):1334-49.

[2] Matthay MA, Zimmerman GA. Acute lung injury and the acute respiratory distress syndrome: four decades of inquiry into pathogenesis and rational management. Am J Respir Cell Mol Biol. 2005 Oct;33(4):319-27.

[3] Rubenfeld GD, Caldwell E, Peabody E, Weaver J, Martin DP, Neff M, et al. Incidence and outcomes of acute lung injury. N Engl J Med. 2005 Oct 20;353(16):1685-93.

[4] Girdhar A, Kumar V, Singh A, Menon B, Vijayan VK. Systemic inflammation and its response to treatment in patients with asthma. Respir Care. 2011 Jun;56(6):800-5.

[5] Jousilahti P, Salomaa V, Hakala K, Rasi V, Vahtera E, Palosuo T. The association of sensitive systemic inflammation markers with bronchial asthma. Ann Allergy Asthma Immunol. 2002 Oct;89(4):381-5.

[6] Olafsdottir IS, Gislason T, Thjodleifsson B, Olafsson I, Gislason D, Jogi R, et al. C reactive protein levels are increased in non-allergic but not allergic asthma: a multicentre epidemiological study. Thorax. 2005 Jun;60(6):451-4.

[7] Takemura M, Matsumoto H, Niimi A, Ueda T, Matsuoka H, Yamaguchi M, et al. High sensitivity C-reactive protein in asthma. Eur Respir J. 2006 May;27(5):908-12.

[8] Wilson CB, Jones PW, O'Leary CJ, Hansell DM, Dowling RB, Cole PJ, et al. Systemic markers of inflammation in stable bronchiectasis. Eur Respir J. 1998 Oct;12(4):820-4.

[9] Martinez-Garcia MA, Perpina-Tordera M, Roman-Sanchez P, Soler-Cataluna JJ, Carratala A, Yago M, et al. [The association between bronchiectasis, systemic inflammation, and tumor necrosis factor alpha]. Arch Bronconeumol. 2008 Jan;44(1):8-14.

[10] Weinrib L, Sharma OP, Quismorio FP, Jr. A long-term study of interstitial lung disease in systemic lupus erythematosus. Semin Arthritis Rheum. 1990 Aug;20(1):48-56.

[11] Hamblin MJ, Horton MR. Rheumatoid arthritis-associated interstitial lung disease: diagnostic dilemma. Pulm Med. 2011;2011:872120.

[12] Fischer A, du Bois R. Interstitial lung disease in connective tissue disorders. Lancet. 2012 Aug 18;380(9842):689-98.

[13] Solomon JJ, Olson AL, Fischer A, Bull T, Brown KK, Raghu G. Scleroderma lung disease. Eur Respir Rev. 2013 Mar 1;22(127):6-19.

[14] Castelino FV, Varga J. Interstitial lung disease in connective tissue diseases: evolving concepts of pathogenesis and management. Arthritis Res Ther. 2010;12(4):213.

[15] Matthay MA, Ware LB, Zimmerman GA. The acute respiratory distress syndrome. J Clin Invest. 2012 Aug 1;122(8):2731-40.

[16] Fry DE. Sepsis syndrome. Am Surg. 2000 Feb;66(2):126-32.

[17] Klune JR, Tsung A. Molecular biology of liver ischemia/reperfusion injury: established mechanisms and recent advancements. Surg Clin North Am. 2010 Aug;90(4): 665-77.

[18] American College of Chest Physicians/Society of Critical Care Medicine Consensus Conference: definitions for sepsis and organ failure and guidelines for the use of innovative therapies in sepsis. Crit Care Med. 1992 Jun;20(6):864-74.

[19] Goris RJ, te Boekhorst TP, Nuytinck JK, Gimbrere JS. Multiple-organ failure. Generalized autodestructive inflammation? Arch Surg. 1985 Oct;120(10):1109-15.

[20] Opitz B, van Laak V, Eitel J, Suttorp N. Innate immune recognition in infectious and noninfectious diseases of the lung. Am J Respir Crit Care Med. 2010 Jun 15;181(12): 1294-309.

[21] Windsor AC, Walsh CJ, Mullen PG, Cook DJ, Fisher BJ, Blocher CR, et al. Tumor necrosis factor-alpha blockade prevents neutrophil CD18 receptor upregulation and attenuates acute lung injury in porcine sepsis without inhibition of neutrophil oxygen radical generation. J Clin Invest. 1993 Apr;91(4):1459-68.

[22] Friedman GD, Klatsky AL, Siegelaub AB. The leukocyte count as a predictor of myocardial infarction. N Engl J Med. 1974 Jun 6;290(23):1275-8.

[23] Grimm RH, Jr., Neaton JD, Ludwig W. Prognostic importance of the white blood cell count for coronary, cancer, and all-cause mortality. JAMA. 1985 Oct 11;254(14): 1932-7.

[24] Weiss ST, Segal MR, Sparrow D, Wager C. Relation of FEV1 and peripheral blood leukocyte count to total mortality. The Normative Aging Study. Am J Epidemiol. 1995 Sep 1;142(5):493-8; discussion 9-503.

[25] Corre F, Lellouch J, Schwartz D. Smoking and leucocyte-counts. Results of an epidemiological survey. Lancet. 1971 Sep 18;2(7725):632-4.

[26] Chan-Yeung M, Abboud R, Buncio AD, Vedal S. Peripheral leucocyte count and longitudinal decline in lung function. Thorax. 1988 Jun;43(6):462-6.

[27] van Eeden SF, Hogg JC. The response of human bone marrow to chronic cigarette smoking. Eur Respir J. 2000 May;15(5):915-21.

[28] Terashima T, Wiggs B, English D, Hogg JC, van Eeden SF. The effect of cigarette smoking on the bone marrow. Am J Respir Crit Care Med. 1997 Mar;155(3):1021-6.

[29] Torres JL, Ridker PM. Clinical use of high sensitivity C-reactive protein for the prediction of adverse cardiovascular events. Curr Opin Cardiol. 2003 Nov;18(6):471-8.

[30] Sin DD, Man SF. Why are patients with chronic obstructive pulmonary disease at increased risk of cardiovascular diseases? The potential role of systemic inflammation in chronic obstructive pulmonary disease. Circulation. 2003 Mar 25;107(11):1514-9.

[31] Shaaban R, Kony S, Driss F, Leynaert B, Soussan D, Pin I, et al. Change in C-reactive protein levels and FEV1 decline: a longitudinal population-based study. Respir Med. 2006 Dec;100(12):2112-20.

[32] Pinto-Plata VM, Mullerova H, Toso JF, Feudjo-Tepie M, Soriano JB, Vessey RS, et al. C-reactive protein in patients with COPD, control smokers and non-smokers. Thorax. 2006 Jan;61(1):23-8.

[33] Sin DD, Lacy P, York E, Man SF. Effects of fluticasone on systemic markers of inflammation in chronic obstructive pulmonary disease. Am J Respir Crit Care Med. 2004 Oct 1;170(7):760-5.

[34] Chung KF. Cytokines in chronic obstructive pulmonary disease. Eur Respir J Suppl. 2001 Dec;34:50s-9s.

[35] Eid AA, Ionescu AA, Nixon LS, Lewis-Jenkins V, Matthews SB, Griffiths TL, et al. Inflammatory response and body composition in chronic obstructive pulmonary disease. Am J Respir Crit Care Med. 2001 Oct 15;164(8 Pt 1):1414-8.

[36] Di Francia M, Barbier D, Mege JL, Orehek J. Tumor necrosis factor-alpha levels and weight loss in chronic obstructive pulmonary disease. Am J Respir Crit Care Med. 1994 Nov;150(5 Pt 1):1453-5.

[37] Gustafsson A, Asman B, Bergstrom K. Cigarette smoking as an aggravating factor in inflammatory tissue-destructive diseases. Increase in tumor necrosis Factor-alpha priming of peripheral neutrophils measured as generation of oxygen radicals. Int J Clin Lab Res. 2000;30(4):187-90.

[38] Noguera A, Batle S, Miralles C, Iglesias J, Busquets X, MacNee W, et al. Enhanced neutrophil response in chronic obstructive pulmonary disease. Thorax. 2001 Jun; 56(6):432-7.

[39] de Godoy I, Donahoe M, Calhoun WJ, Mancino J, Rogers RM. Elevated TNF-alpha production by peripheral blood monocytes of weight-losing COPD patients. Am J Respir Crit Care Med. 1996 Feb;153(2):633-7.

[40] Schols AM, Buurman WA, Staal van den Brekel AJ, Dentener MA, Wouters EF. Evidence for a relation between metabolic derangements and increased levels of inflammatory mediators in a subgroup of patients with chronic obstructive pulmonary disease. Thorax. 1996 Aug;51(8):819-24.

[41] Dentener MA, Creutzberg EC, Schols AM, Mantovani A, van't Veer C, Buurman WA, et al. Systemic anti-inflammatory mediators in COPD: increase in soluble interleukin 1 receptor II during treatment of exacerbations. Thorax. 2001 Sep;56(9):721-6.

[42] Terashima T, Wiggs B, English D, Hogg JC, van Eeden SF. Phagocytosis of small carbon particles (PM10) by alveolar macrophages stimulates the release of polymorphonuclear leukocytes from bone marrow. Am J Respir Crit Care Med. 1997 Apr;155(4): 1441-7.

[43] Mukae H, Vincent R, Quinlan K, English D, Hards J, Hogg JC, et al. The effect of repeated exposure to particulate air pollution (PM10) on the bone marrow. Am J Respir Crit Care Med. 2001 Jan;163(1):201-9.

[44] Tan WC, Qiu D, Liam BL, Ng TP, Lee SH, van Eeden SF, et al. The human bone marrow response to acute air pollution caused by forest fires. Am J Respir Crit Care Med. 2000 Apr;161(4 Pt 1):1213-7.

[45] van Eeden SF, Tan WC, Suwa T, Mukae H, Terashima T, Fujii T, et al. Cytokines involved in the systemic inflammatory response induced by exposure to particulate matter air pollutants (PM(10)). Am J Respir Crit Care Med. 2001 Sep 1;164(5):826-30.

[46] Vincent R, Bjarnason SG, Adamson IY, Hedgecock C, Kumarathasan P, Guenette J, et al. Acute pulmonary toxicity of urban particulate matter and ozone. Am J Pathol. 1997 Dec;151(6):1563-70.

[47] Fujii T, Hayashi S, Hogg JC, Vincent R, Van Eeden SF. Particulate matter induces cytokine expression in human bronchial epithelial cells. Am J Respir Cell Mol Biol. 2001 Sep;25(3):265-71.

[48] Boland S, Baeza-Squiban A, Fournier T, Houcine O, Gendron MC, Chevrier M, et al. Diesel exhaust particles are taken up by human airway epithelial cells in vitro and alter cytokine production. Am J Physiol. 1999 Apr;276(4 Pt 1):L604-13.

[49] Hashimoto S, Gon Y, Matsumoto K, Takeshita I, Maruoka S, Horie T. Inhalant corticosteroids inhibit hyperosmolarity-induced, and cooling and rewarming-induced interleukin-8 and RANTES production by human bronchial epithelial cells. Am J Respir Crit Care Med. 2000 Sep;162(3 Pt 1):1075-80.

[50] Fujii T, Hayashi S, Hogg JC, Mukae H, Suwa T, Goto Y, et al. Interaction of alveolar macrophages and airway epithelial cells following exposure to particulate matter produces mediators that stimulate the bone marrow. Am J Respir Cell Mol Biol. 2002 Jul;27(1):34-41.

[51] Al Lawati N, Mulgrew A, Cheema R, vanEeden S, Butt A, Fleetham J, et al. Pro-atherogenic cytokine profile of patients with suspected obstructive sleep apnea. Sleep Breath. 2009 Nov;13(4):391-5.

[52] Bruno A, Alessi M, Soresi S, Bonanno A, Riccobono L, Montalbano AM, et al. Increased leptin/leptin receptor pathway affects systemic and airway inflammation in COPD former smokers. J Inflamm Res. 2011;4:51-9.

[53] Bijanzadeh M, Ramachandra NB, Mahesh PA, Savitha MR, Vijayakumar GS, Kumar P, et al. Soluble intercellular adhesion molecule-1 and E-selectin in patients with asthma exacerbation. Lung. 2009 Sep-Oct;187(5):315-20.

[54] Friedman J, Goldberg H, Horvath TB, Meares RA. The effect of tobacco smoking on evoked potentials. Clin Exp Pharmacol Physiol. 1974 May-Jun;1(3):249-58.

[55] Friedman J, Horvath T, Meares R. Tobacco smoking and a 'stimulus barrier'. Nature. 1974 Mar 29;248(447):455-6.

[56] van Eeden SF, Granton J, Hards JM, Moore B, Hogg JC. Expression of the cell adhesion molecules on leukocytes that demarginate during acute maximal exercise. J Appl Physiol. 1999 Mar;86(3):970-6.

[57] Terashima T, Amakawa K, Matsumaru A, van Eeden S, Hogg JC, Yamaguchi K. BAL induces an increase in peripheral blood neutrophils and cytokine levels in healthy volunteers and patients with pneumonia. Chest. 2001 Jun;119(6):1724-9.

[58] Muchmore HG, Blackburn AB, Shurley JT, Pierce CM, McKown BA. Neutropenia in healthy men at the South Polar Plateau. Arch Intern Med. 1970 Apr;125(4):646-8.

[59] Sakai M, Sato Y, Sato S, Ihara S, Onizuka M, Sakakibara Y, et al. Effect of relocating to areas of reduced atmospheric particulate matter levels on the human circulating leukocyte count. J Appl Physiol. 2004 Nov;97(5):1774-80.

[60] Bicknell S, van Eeden S, Hayashi S, Hards J, English D, Hogg JC. A non-radioisotopic method for tracing neutrophils in vivo using 5'-bromo-2'-deoxyuridine. Am J Respir Cell Mol Biol. 1994 Jan;10(1):16-23.

[61] Terashima T, Wiggs B, English D, Hogg JC, van Eeden SF. Polymorphonuclear leukocyte transit times in bone marrow during streptococcal pneumonia. Am J Physiol. 1996 Oct;271(4 Pt 1):L587-92.

[62] Goto Y, Hogg JC, Suwa T, Quinlan KB, van Eeden SF. A novel method to quantify the turnover and release of monocytes from the bone marrow using the thymidine analog 5'-bromo-2'-deoxyuridine. Am J Physiol Cell Physiol. 2003 Aug;285(2):C253-9.

[63] Terashima T, Klut ME, English D, Hards J, Hogg JC, van Eeden SF. Cigarette smoking causes sequestration of polymorphonuclear leukocytes released from the bone marrow in lung microvessels. Am J Respir Cell Mol Biol. 1999 Jan;20(1):171-7.

[64] Goto Y, Hogg JC, Shih CH, Ishii H, Vincent R, van Eeden SF. Exposure to ambient particles accelerates monocyte release from bone marrow in atherosclerotic rabbits. Am J Physiol Lung Cell Mol Physiol. 2004 Jul;287(1):L79-85.

[65] Lawrence E, Van Eeden S, English D, Hogg JC. Polymorphonuclear leukocyte (PMN) migration in streptococcal pneumonia: comparison of older PMN with those recently released from the marrow. Am J Respir Cell Mol Biol. 1996 Mar;14(3):217-24.

[66] van Eeden SF, Kitagawa Y, Sato Y, Hogg JC. Polymorphonuclear leukocytes released from the bone marrow and acute lung injury. Chest. 1999 Jul;116(1 Suppl):43S-6S.

[67] van Eeden SF, Lawrence E, Sato Y, Kitagawa Y, Hogg JC. Neutrophils released from the bone marrow by granulocyte colony-stimulating factor sequester in lung microvessels but are slow to migrate. Eur Respir J. 2000 Jun;15(6):1079-86.

[68] Gabay C, Kushner I. Acute-phase proteins and other systemic responses to inflammation. N Engl J Med. 1999 Feb 11;340(6):448-54.

[69] Heinrich J, Assmann G. Fibrinogen and cardiovascular risk. J Cardiovasc Risk. 1995 Jun;2(3):197-205.

[70] Haverkate F, Thompson SG, Pyke SD, Gallimore JR, Pepys MB. Production of C-reactive protein and risk of coronary events in stable and unstable angina. European Concerted Action on Thrombosis and Disabilities Angina Pectoris Study Group. Lancet. 1997 Feb 15;349(9050):462-6.

[71] Tracy RP, Lemaitre RN, Psaty BM, Ives DG, Evans RW, Cushman M, et al. Relationship of C-reactive protein to risk of cardiovascular disease in the elderly. Results from the Cardiovascular Health Study and the Rural Health Promotion Project. Arterioscler Thromb Vasc Biol. 1997 Jun;17(6):1121-7.

[72] Ridker PM, Cushman M, Stampfer MJ, Tracy RP, Hennekens CH. Inflammation, aspirin, and the risk of cardiovascular disease in apparently healthy men. N Engl J Med. 1997 Apr 3;336(14):973-9.

[73] Ridker PM, Buring JE, Shih J, Matias M, Hennekens CH. Prospective study of C-reactive protein and the risk of future cardiovascular events among apparently healthy women. Circulation. 1998 Aug 25;98(8):731-3.

[74] Mire-Sluis A, Thorpe R. Quality considerations for recombinant DNA-derived biological therapeutic products: a control perspective on cytokines. BioDrugs. 1999 Jun; 11(6):367-76.

[75] Topham MK, Carveth HJ, McIntyre TM, Prescott SM, Zimmerman GA. Human endothelial cells regulate polymorphonuclear leukocyte degranulation. FASEB J. 1998 Jun;12(9):733-46.

[76] Mire-Sluis AR. Analytical characterisation of cytokines and growth factors. Dev Biol Stand. 1999;97:3-9.

[77] Mackiewicz A, Laciak M, Gorny A, Baumann H. Leukemia inhibitory factor, interferon gamma and dexamethasone regulate N-glycosylation of alpha 1-protease inhibitor in human hepatoma cells. Eur J Cell Biol. 1993 Apr;60(2):331-6.

[78] Suwa T, Hogg JC, Klut ME, Hards J, van Eeden SF. Interleukin-6 changes deformability of neutrophils and induces their sequestration in the lung. Am J Respir Crit Care Med. 2001 Mar;163(4):970-6.

[79] Schaaf BM, Boehmke F, Esnaashari H, Seitzer U, Kothe H, Maass M, et al. Pneumococcal septic shock is associated with the interleukin-10-1082 gene promoter polymorphism. Am J Respir Crit Care Med. 2003 Aug 15;168(4):476-80.

[80] Shu Q, Fang X, Chen Q, Stuber F. IL-10 polymorphism is associated with increased incidence of severe sepsis. Chin Med J (Engl). 2003 Nov;116(11):1756-9.

[81] Rautou PE, Vion AC, Amabile N, Chironi G, Simon A, Tedgui A, et al. Microparticles, vascular function, and atherothrombosis. Circ Res. 2011 Aug 19;109(5):593-606.

[82] Mause SF, Weber C. Microparticles: protagonists of a novel communication network for intercellular information exchange. Circ Res. 2010 Oct 29;107(9):1047-57.

[83] Choi HS, Ashitate Y, Lee JH, Kim SH, Matsui A, Insin N, et al. Rapid translocation of nanoparticles from the lung airspaces to the body. Nat Biotechnol. 2010 Dec;28(12):1300-3.

[84] Oberdorster G, Sharp Z, Atudorei V, Elder A, Gelein R, Lunts A, et al. Extrapulmonary translocation of ultrafine carbon particles following whole-body inhalation exposure of rats. J Toxicol Environ Health A. 2002 Oct 25;65(20):1531-43.

[85] Morel O, Jesel L, Freyssinet JM, Toti F. Cellular mechanisms underlying the formation of circulating microparticles. Arterioscler Thromb Vasc Biol. 2011 Jan;31(1):15-26.

[86] Amabile N, Rautou PE, Tedgui A, Boulanger CM. Microparticles: key protagonists in cardiovascular disorders. Semin Thromb Hemost. 2010 Nov;36(8):907-16.

[87] Boulanger CM, Amabile N, Tedgui A. Circulating microparticles: a potential prognostic marker for atherosclerotic vascular disease. Hypertension. 2006 Aug;48(2):180-6.

[88] Boulanger CM, Scoazec A, Ebrahimian T, Henry P, Mathieu E, Tedgui A, et al. Circulating microparticles from patients with myocardial infarction cause endothelial dysfunction. Circulation. 2001 Nov 27;104(22):2649-52.

[89] Thomashow MA, Shimbo D, Parikh MA, Hoffman EA, Vogel-Claussen J, Hueper K, et al. Endothelial microparticles in mild chronic obstructive pulmonary disease and emphysema. The Multi-Ethnic Study of Atherosclerosis Chronic Obstructive Pulmonary Disease study. Am J Respir Crit Care Med. 2013 Jul 1;188(1):60-8.

[90] Takahashi T, Kobayashi S, Fujino N, Suzuki T, Ota C, He M, et al. Increased circulating endothelial microparticles in COPD patients: a potential biomarker for COPD exacerbation susceptibility. Thorax. 2012 Dec;67(12):1067-74.

[91] Guiducci S, Distler JH, Jungel A, Huscher D, Huber LC, Michel BA, et al. The relationship between plasma microparticles and disease manifestations in patients with systemic sclerosis. Arthritis Rheum. 2008 Sep;58(9):2845-53.

[92] van Eeden SF, de Beer P. Community-acquired pneumonia: evidence of functional inactivation of alpha 1 proteinase inhibitor. Crit Care Med. 1990 Nov;18(11):1204-9.

[93] Tamagawa E, Suda K, Wei Y, Xing L, Mui T, Li Y, et al. Endotoxin-induced translocation of interleukin-6 from lungs to the systemic circulation. Innate Immun. 2009 Aug;15(4):251-8.

[94] Kido T, Tamagawa E, Bai N, Suda K, Yang HH, Li Y, et al. Particulate matter induces translocation of IL-6 from the lung to the systemic circulation. Am J Respir Cell Mol Biol. 2011 Feb;44(2):197-204.

[95] Godleski JJ, Verrier RL, Koutrakis P, Catalano P, Coull B, Reinisch U, et al. Mechanisms of morbidity and mortality from exposure to ambient air particles. Res Rep Health Eff Inst. 2000 Feb(91):5-88; discussion 9-103.

[96] Nemmar A, Hoet PH, Vanquickenborne B, Dinsdale D, Thomeer M, Hoylaerts MF, et al. Passage of inhaled particles into the blood circulation in humans. Circulation. 2002 Jan 29;105(4):411-4.

[97] Peters A, Veronesi B, Calderon-Garciduenas L, Gehr P, Chen LC, Geiser M, et al. Translocation and potential neurological effects of fine and ultrafine particles a critical update. Part Fibre Toxicol. 2006;3:13.

[98] Fry DE. Sepsis, systemic inflammatory response, and multiple organ dysfunction: the mystery continues. Am Surg. 2012 Jan;78(1):1-8.

[99] Suwa T, Hogg JC, Quinlan KB, Ohgami A, Vincent R, van Eeden SF. Particulate air pollution induces progression of atherosclerosis. J Am Coll Cardiol. 2002 Mar 20;39(6):935-42.

[100] Sun Q, Wang A, Jin X, Natanzon A, Duquaine D, Brook RD, et al. Long-term air pollution exposure and acceleration of atherosclerosis and vascular inflammation in an animal model. JAMA. 2005 Dec 21;294(23):3003-10.

[101] Yatera K, Hsieh J, Hogg JC, Tranfield E, Suzuki H, Shih CH, et al. Particulate matter air pollution exposure promotes recruitment of monocytes into atherosclerotic plaques. Am J Physiol Heart Circ Physiol. 2008 Feb;294(2):H944-53.

[102] Tamagawa E, Bai N, Morimoto K, Gray C, Mui T, Yatera K, et al. Particulate matter exposure induces persistent lung inflammation and endothelial dysfunction. Am J Physiol Lung Cell Mol Physiol. 2008 Jul;295(1):L79-85.

[103] van Eeden SF, Sin DD. Chronic obstructive pulmonary disease: a chronic systemic inflammatory disease. Respiration. 2008;75(2):224-38.

[104] Gan WQ, Man SF, Senthilselvan A, Sin DD. Association between chronic obstructive pulmonary disease and systemic inflammation: a systematic review and a meta-analysis. Thorax. 2004 Jul;59(7):574-80.

[105] Wedzicha JA, Seemungal TA, MacCallum PK, Paul EA, Donaldson GC, Bhowmik A, et al. Acute exacerbations of chronic obstructive pulmonary disease are accompanied by elevations of plasma fibrinogen and serum IL-6 levels. Thromb Haemost. 2000 Aug;84(2):210-5.

[106] Karadag F, Karul AB, Cildag O, Yilmaz M, Ozcan H. Biomarkers of systemic inflammation in stable and exacerbation phases of COPD. Lung. 2008 Nov-Dec;186(6):403-9.

[107] Sin DD, Wu L, Man SF. The relationship between reduced lung function and cardiovascular mortality: a population-based study and a systematic review of the literature. Chest. 2005 Jun;127(6):1952-9.

[108] Engelhart MJ, Geerlings MI, Meijer J, Kiliaan A, Ruitenberg A, van Swieten JC, et al. Inflammatory proteins in plasma and the risk of dementia: the rotterdam study. Arch Neurol. 2004 May;61(5):668-72.

[109] Borson S, Scanlan J, Friedman S, Zuhr E, Fields J, Aylward E, et al. Modeling the impact of COPD on the brain. Int J Chron Obstruct Pulmon Dis. 2008;3(3):429-34.

[110] Agusti A, Morla M, Sauleda J, Saus C, Busquets X. NF-kappaB activation and iNOS upregulation in skeletal muscle of patients with COPD and low body weight. Thorax. 2004 Jun;59(6):483-7.

[111] Agusti AG, Sauleda J, Miralles C, Gomez C, Togores B, Sala E, et al. Skeletal muscle apoptosis and weight loss in chronic obstructive pulmonary disease. Am J Respir Crit Care Med. 2002 Aug 15;166(4):485-9.

[112] Schols AM, Slangen J, Volovics L, Wouters EF. Weight loss is a reversible factor in the prognosis of chronic obstructive pulmonary disease. Am J Respir Crit Care Med. 1998 Jun;157(6 Pt 1):1791-7.

[113] Agusti AG. Systemic effects of chronic obstructive pulmonary disease. Proc Am Thorac Soc. 2005;2(4):367-70; discussion 71-2.

[114] Biskobing DM. COPD and osteoporosis. Chest. 2002 Feb;121(2):609-20.

[115] Rana JS, Mittleman MA, Sheikh J, Hu FB, Manson JE, Colditz GA, et al. Chronic obstructive pulmonary disease, asthma, and risk of type 2 diabetes in women. Diabetes Care. 2004 Oct;27(10):2478-84.

[116] Fahy JV. Eosinophilic and neutrophilic inflammation in asthma: insights from clinical studies. Proc Am Thorac Soc. 2009 May 1;6(3):256-9.

[117] Warwick G, Thomas PS, Yates DH. Non-invasive biomarkers in exacerbations of obstructive lung disease. Respirology. 2013 Jul;18(5):874-84.

[118] Kato M, Yamada Y, Maruyama K, Hayashi Y. Serum eosinophil cationic protein and 27 cytokines/chemokines in acute exacerbation of childhood asthma. Int Arch Allergy Immunol. 2010;152 Suppl 1:62-6.

[119] Martinet Y, Rom WN, Grotendorst GR, Martin GR, Crystal RG. Exaggerated spontaneous release of platelet-derived growth factor by alveolar macrophages from patients with idiopathic pulmonary fibrosis. N Engl J Med. 1987 Jul 23;317(4):202-9.

[120] Wynn TA. Integrating mechanisms of pulmonary fibrosis. J Exp Med. 2011 Jul 4;208(7):1339-50.

[121] Doi K, Ishizu T, Fujita T, Noiri E. Lung injury following acute kidney injury: kidney-lung crosstalk. Clin Exp Nephrol. 2011 Aug;15(4):464-70.

[122] Quilez ME, Lopez-Aguilar J, Blanch L. Organ crosstalk during acute lung injury, acute respiratory distress syndrome, and mechanical ventilation. Curr Opin Crit Care. 2012 Feb;18(1):23-8.

[123] Ahuja N, Andres-Hernando A, Altmann C, Bhargava R, Bacalja J, Webb RG, et al. Circulating IL-6 mediates lung injury via CXCL1 production after acute kidney injury in mice. Am J Physiol Renal Physiol. 2012 Sep 15;303(6):F864-72.

[124] Zhang H, Neuhofer P, Song L, Rabe B, Lesina M, Kurkowski MU, et al. IL-6 trans-signaling promotes pancreatitis-associated lung injury and lethality. J Clin Invest. 2013 Mar 1;123(3):1019-31.

[125] Klut ME, Doerschuk CM, Van Eeden SF, Burns AR, Hogg JC. Activation of neutrophils within pulmonary microvessels of rabbits exposed to cigarette smoke. Am J Respir Cell Mol Biol. 1993 Jul;9(1):82-9.

[126] Klut ME, van Eeden SF, Whalen BA, Verburgt LM, English D, Hogg JC. Neutrophil activation and lung injury associated with chronic endotoxemia in rabbits. Exp Lung Res. 1996 Jul-Aug;22(4):449-65.

[127] Lang JD, Hickman-Davis JM. One-hit, two-hit... is there really any benefit? Clin Exp Immunol. 2005 Aug;141(2):211-4.

[128] Lee JS, Su X, Rackley C, Matthay MA, Gupta N. Priming with endotoxin increases acute lung injury in mice by enhancing the severity of lung endothelial injury. Anat Rec (Hoboken). 2011 Jan;294(1):165-72.

[129] Sato Y, van Eeden SF, English D, Hogg JC. Bacteremic pneumococcal pneumonia: bone marrow release and pulmonary sequestration of neutrophils. Crit Care Med. 1998 Mar;26(3):501-9.

[130] Sato Y, Van Eeden SF, English D, Hogg JC. Pulmonary sequestration of polymorphonuclear leukocytes released from bone marrow in bacteremic infection. Am J Physiol. 1998 Aug;275(2 Pt 1):L255-61.

[131] Hogg JC. Why does airway inflammation persist after the smoking stops? Thorax. 2006 Feb;61(2):96-7.

[132] Carlsten C, Dybuncio A, Pui MM, Chan-Yeung M. Respiratory impairment and systemic inflammation in cedar asthmatics removed from exposure. PLoS One. 2013;8(2):e57166.

[133] Eichacker PQ, Parent C, Kalil A, Esposito C, Cui X, Banks SM, et al. Risk and the efficacy of antiinflammatory agents: retrospective and confirmatory studies of sepsis. Am J Respir Crit Care Med. 2002 Nov 1;166(9):1197-205.

[134] Rennard SI, Fogarty C, Kelsen S, Long W, Ramsdell J, Allison J, et al. The safety and efficacy of infliximab in moderate to severe chronic obstructive pulmonary disease. Am J Respir Crit Care Med. 2007 May 1;175(9):926-34.

[135] Buff SM, Yu H, McCall JN, Caldwell SM, Ferkol TW, Flotte TR, et al. IL-10 delivery by AAV5 vector attenuates inflammation in mice with Pseudomonas pneumonia. Gene Ther. 2010 May;17(5):567-76.

[136] Sawa T, Corry DB, Gropper MA, Ohara M, Kurahashi K, Wiener-Kronish JP. IL-10 improves lung injury and survival in Pseudomonas aeruginosa pneumonia. J Immunol. 1997 Sep 15;159(6):2858-66.

[137] Zuany-Amorim C, Haile S, Leduc D, Dumarey C, Huerre M, Vargaftig BB, et al. Interleukin-10 inhibits antigen-induced cellular recruitment into the airways of sensitized mice. J Clin Invest. 1995 Jun;95(6):2644-51.

[138] Dokka S, Malanga CJ, Shi X, Chen F, Castranova V, Rojanasakul Y. Inhibition of endotoxin-induced lung inflammation by interleukin-10 gene transfer in mice. Am J Physiol Lung Cell Mol Physiol. 2000 Nov;279(5):L872-7.

[139] Serhan CN. Novel lipid mediators and resolution mechanisms in acute inflammation: to resolve or not? Am J Pathol. 2010 Oct;177(4):1576-91.

[140] Hsiao HM, Sapinoro RE, Thatcher TH, Croasdell A, Levy EP, Fulton RA, et al. A novel anti-inflammatory and pro-resolving role for resolvin D1 in acute cigarette smoke-induced lung inflammation. PLoS One. 2013;8(3):e58258.

[141] Shahar E, Folsom AR, Melnick SL, Tockman MS, Comstock GW, Gennaro V, et al. Dietary n-3 polyunsaturated fatty acids and smoking-related chronic obstructive pulmonary disease. Atherosclerosis Risk in Communities Study Investigators. N Engl J Med. 1994 Jul 28;331(4):228-33.

[142] Jain MK, Ridker PM. Anti-inflammatory effects of statins: clinical evidence and basic mechanisms. Nat Rev Drug Discov. 2005 Dec;4(12):977-87.

[143] Zhou Q, Liao JK. Pleiotropic effects of statins. - Basic research and clinical perspectives. Circ J. 2010 May;74(5):818-26.

[144] Laufs U, Liao JK. Isoprenoid metabolism and the pleiotropic effects of statins. Curr Atheroscler Rep. 2003 Sep;5(5):372-8.

[145] Naidu BV, Woolley SM, Farivar AS, Thomas R, Fraga C, Mulligan MS. Simvastatin ameliorates injury in an experimental model of lung ischemia-reperfusion. J Thorac Cardiovasc Surg. 2003 Aug;126(2):482-9.

[146] Fischetti F, Carretta R, Borotto G, Durigutto P, Bulla R, Meroni PL, et al. Fluvastatin treatment inhibits leucocyte adhesion and extravasation in models of complement-mediated acute inflammation. Clin Exp Immunol. 2004 Feb;135(2):186-93.

[147] Jacobson JR, Barnard JW, Grigoryev DN, Ma SF, Tuder RM, Garcia JG. Simvastatin attenuates vascular leak and inflammation in murine inflammatory lung injury. Am J Physiol Lung Cell Mol Physiol. 2005 Jun;288(6):L1026-32.

[148] Miyata R, Bai N, Vincent R, Sin DD, Van Eeden SF. Novel properties of statins: suppression of the systemic and bone marrow responses induced by exposure to ambi-

ent particulate matter (PM(10)) air pollution. Am J Physiol Lung Cell Mol Physiol. 2012 Sep 15;303(6):L492-9.

[149] Miyata R, Bai N, Vincent R, Sin DD, Van Eeden SF. Statins reduce ambient particulate matter-induced lung inflammation by promoting the clearance of particulate matter, < 10 mum from lung tissues. Chest. 2013 Feb 1;143(2):452-60.

[150] Chalmers JD, Singanayagam A, Murray MP, Hill AT. Prior statin use is associated with improved outcomes in community-acquired pneumonia. Am J Med. 2008 Nov; 121(11):1002-7 e1.

[151] Mortensen EM, Restrepo MI, Anzueto A, Pugh J. The effect of prior statin use on 30-day mortality for patients hospitalized with community-acquired pneumonia. Respir Res. 2005;6:82.

[152] Thomsen RW, Riis A, Kornum JB, Christensen S, Johnsen SP, Sorensen HT. Preadmission use of statins and outcomes after hospitalization with pneumonia: population-based cohort study of 29,900 patients. Arch Intern Med. 2008 Oct 27;168(19): 2081-7.

[153] Blamoun AI, Batty GN, DeBari VA, Rashid AO, Sheikh M, Khan MA. Statins may reduce episodes of exacerbation and the requirement for intubation in patients with COPD: evidence from a retrospective cohort study. Int J Clin Pract. 2008 Sep;62(9): 1373-8.

[154] Frost FJ, Petersen H, Tollestrup K, Skipper B. Influenza and COPD mortality protection as pleiotropic, dose-dependent effects of statins. Chest. 2007 Apr;131(4):1006-12.

[155] Ishida W, Kajiwara T, Ishii M, Fujiwara F, Taneichi H, Takebe N, et al. Decrease in mortality rate of chronic obstructive pulmonary disease (COPD) with statin use: a population-based analysis in Japan. Tohoku J Exp Med. 2007 Jul;212(3):265-73.

[156] Keddissi JI, Younis WG, Chbeir EA, Daher NN, Dernaika TA, Kinasewitz GT. The use of statins and lung function in current and former smokers. Chest. 2007 Dec; 132(6):1764-71.

[157] Lee TM, Lin MS, Chang NC. Usefulness of C-reactive protein and interleukin-6 as predictors of outcomes in patients with chronic obstructive pulmonary disease receiving pravastatin. Am J Cardiol. 2008 Feb 15;101(4):530-5.

[158] Mancini GB, Etminan M, Zhang B, Levesque LE, FitzGerald JM, Brophy JM. Reduction of morbidity and mortality by statins, angiotensin-converting enzyme inhibitors, and angiotensin receptor blockers in patients with chronic obstructive pulmonary disease. J Am Coll Cardiol. 2006 Jun 20;47(12):2554-60.

[159] Soyseth V, Brekke PH, Smith P, Omland T. Statin use is associated with reduced mortality in COPD. Eur Respir J. 2007 Feb;29(2):279-83.

[160] Melbye H, Halvorsen DS, Hartz I, Medbo A, Brox J, Eggen AE, et al. Bronchial airflow limitation, smoking, body mass index, and statin use are strongly associated

with the C-reactive protein level in the elderly. The Tromso Study 2001. Respir Med. 2007 Dec;101(12):2541-9.

[161] van Gestel YR, Hoeks SE, Sin DD, Simsek C, Welten GM, Schouten O, et al. Effect of statin therapy on mortality in patients with peripheral arterial disease and comparison of those with versus without associated chronic obstructive pulmonary disease. Am J Cardiol. 2008 Jul 15;102(2):192-6.

[162] van Eeden SF, Hogg JC. Systemic inflammatory response induced by particulate matter air pollution: the importance of bone-marrow stimulation. J Toxicol Environ Health A. 2002 Oct 25;65(20):1597-613.

[163] Stary HC, Chandler AB, Dinsmore RE, Fuster V, Glagov S, Insull W, Jr., et al. A definition of advanced types of atherosclerotic lesions and a histological classification of atherosclerosis. A report from the Committee on Vascular Lesions of the Council on Arteriosclerosis, American Heart Association. Circulation. 1995 Sep 1;92(5):1355-74.

[164] Stary HC, Chandler AB, Glagov S, Guyton JR, Insull W, Jr., Rosenfeld ME, et al. A definition of initial, fatty streak, and intermediate lesions of atherosclerosis. A report from the Committee on Vascular Lesions of the Council on Arteriosclerosis, American Heart Association. Circulation. 1994 May;89(5):2462-78.

[165] Guidelines for the evaluation of impairment/disability in patients with asthma. American Thoracic Society. Medical Section of the American Lung Association. Am Rev Respir Dis. 1993 Apr;147(4):1056-61.